Go Go Yoga for Kids: Yoga Lessons for Children

Teaching Yoga to Children Through Poses, Breathing Exercises, Games, and Stories

By Sara J. Weis

Find your free Yoga Pose Bingo Cards

www.gogoyogakids.com/bingo

Any physical activity has some risk of injury. Please be aware of your own limits as well as your student's limits.

This book is dedicated to all the children who inspire me every day, and especially to my own three, Megan, Lucy and Max.

Table of Contents

Preface 1

Introduction 4

Chapter 1: The Benefits of Yoga for Children 6

Chapter 2: Secrets to Teaching Yoga to Children 8

Chapter 3: Let's Get Started 12

Chapter 4: Begin with Breath 15

Chapter 5: How to Introduce Yoga Poses to Children 18

Chapter 6: Kids Yoga Games 21

Chapter 7: Top 12 Props to Use in Teaching Kids Yoga 35

Chapter 8. Building Mindfulness in Children Through Moving
Meditation and Mantras 40

Chapter 9: Introduction to Kids Yoga Lesson Planning 47

Chapter 10: Lesson Plans 50

Chapter 11: Quick and Easy No-Time-to-Plan Kids Yoga
Lesson..107

Chapter 12: Read Aloud Books for Yoga and Movement 111

Chapter 13: Pose Glossary 139

Index..152

Preface

When I first tried yoga many years ago, I knew immediately that it was a perfect fit for myself and what I needed both mentally and physically. Before my discovery, though, I was in the midst of living a very busy and scheduled life. I didn't take any time to myself to be in the moment, breathe and move my body mindfully.

Teaching elementary school, working on my master's degree, and raising three young children kept me on the go. As one who is always eager to try new things, I was also training for marathons and triathlons and never missed my workouts or early morning training sessions.

As one can imagine, all of this began to take a toll on my mind and body. I was stronger than I ever had been on the outside, but sleepless nights, anxiety, and nagging pain were all there on the inside. During my last half marathon, a labral tear in my hip brought my long-distance running days to an end.

I could still run, but it wasn't the same. I didn't have the same desire to push myself as hard. As I slowed down, literally, I realized I needed to make some changes. Wanting to remain active and fit, I decided to try an alternative workout and showed up for a yoga class at my local gym.

I fell in love with yoga during my very first class. It filled in everything that had been missing in my body and mind. I loved learning all of the poses and recognizing how they made me feel. I appreciated the deep breathing, twists, and detoxing. Yoga brought me the sense of strength, balance, flexibility, and focus that I needed. My body began to heal and my mind calmed.

Being a teacher and mother, I wanted right away to share my discovery of yoga with all the kids in my life. I realized that if they could have some of the same knowledge, techniques, and skills that I now had, it could make a big impact on their health and well-being.

Eager to get started, I searched everywhere for kids yoga resources such as games, lesson plans, and child-approved yoga activities, only to find that most of what was available was not very age appropriate or engaging. Frustrated with the lack of resources, I went into full-blown lesson plan writing. The teacher in me came out in full strength. I took the things kids are interested in such as animals, super heroes, and adventure and then created corresponding yoga poses and games that were kid-friendly and engaging.

Before long I began teaching kids yoga classes in schools, preschools, daycares, clubs, camps, and at yoga-themed birthday parties. The kids I taught loved these themed yoga lesson plans and games. For me, it was enjoyable and rewarding to make yoga relevant and fun for kids. I loved that they were getting introduced to yoga at such young ages.

After leading hundreds of classes and instructing thousands of children, I knew I really wanted to share with others all that I'd learned and developed. *Go Go Yoga for Kids: A Complete Guide to Using Yoga with Kids* was published, and soon after that, the *Kids Yoga Challenge Pose Cards* were created as a companion to the book. Since then, my interest in yoga for kids and its accompanying benefits has continued to grow.

To help others gain confidence in introducing kids to yoga, I have also developed two online kids yoga teacher training classes: **Kids Yoga 101: How to Teach Yoga to Kids** and also **Teaching Kids Yoga at School and Home**.

Thank you for joining me in this adventure and for sharing yoga and all its benefits with the kids in your life.

Namaste,

Sara

Introduction

Are you a parent looking for yoga poses and activities to do with your children at home?

Are you a teacher looking for easy and creative ways to integrate yoga and mindfulness into your curriculum?

Are you a children's yoga instructor looking for new ideas to incorporate into your yoga classes?

Are you a counselor or health care professional or someone else who works with children and wants to help them learn how to increase their concentration, self-control, and self-confidence while also learning stress management skills?

Go Go Yoga for Kids offers all the tools and resources you need to introduce yoga to children at a whole new level.

Welcome! I'm Sara Weis, and I am excited to help you become comfortable with teaching yoga for kids in fun, effective, and memorable ways. As a school teacher and kids yoga instructor for many years, I have gained a lot of experience and knowledge on the best practices for using yoga with kids. Because yoga has so many mental and physical benefits for children, both now and throughout their lives, I am passionate about introducing children to yoga. That is why I have been sure to include many ideas and resources to help you introduce children to yoga through movement, poses, games, mindfulness and more.

Over the years I have taught hundreds of kids yoga classes, instructed thousands of children, and led many kids yoga workshops and presentations for school teachers, parents, children's yoga instructors, and counselors. While working with many different ages in a variety of settings, I have created engaging kids yoga lesson plans that will be of help to anyone who wants to confidently and effectively introduce yoga to children.

When I first started teaching kids yoga, every one of the children's yoga classes I taught required a lot of planning on my part. Admittedly, it took me hours to create a single kids yoga class. After all, I needed to come up with a theme and relevant yoga poses, plan a breathing exercise, find a quality picture book, plan appropriate music, create engaging yoga games to practice the poses, plus build in mindfulness and team building. It was so much! As a teacher and not one to "wing it," I had to make sure the lesson plans were complete and organized from beginning to end and also that they included the opportunity to possibly integrate it into a school curriculum. As a mom, I have made sure the lesson plans are relevant and engaging for a home practice with kids.

Since kids, teaching, and yoga are my passions, my goal has been to take the guesswork out of teaching yoga to children. I want to help you be more efficient, organized, professional, and inspired, so you can absolutely have fun while introducing yoga to kids.

Chapter 1: The Benefits of Yoga for Children

Children receive many benefits from being introduced to yoga. Introducing children to yoga at an early age can help them learn healthy lifestyle habits and set the foundation for a fit future. Teaching yoga to children opens the door to a practice that nurtures healthy bodies, minds, and spirits. A few of the primary benefits are listed below. The good news is the benefits are not just for kids. When you teach yoga to children, you are not only giving them lifelong skills and benefits, but you are also receiving them yourself.

Increases Flexibility and Balance

Did you know that your flexibility and balance start to decrease after age seven? Fortunately, by practicing yoga poses children and adults can maintain and improve in both of these areas.

As you teach yoga to children, please remember that they do not need to have perfect alignment with the poses. Do not get hung up on the knee being at a perfect right angle or if everyone looks exactly like the illustration. Yoga is not about perfection. Everyone's body is different, and it is always changing. The important matter is that children are being introduced to beneficial poses as their bodies grow and change.

Improves Concentration and Focus

As adults we know that children need to be able to concentrate and focus. But the continued and frequent use of phones, tablets, and other devices means kids are becoming accustomed to immediate gratification. Yoga poses and breathing exercises help teach children how to wait and be still.

Be More Present and Mindful

Adults and kids have become accustomed to a fast-paced lifestyle. We tend to move quickly from one thing to another without truly appreciating the moment we are presently in. Yoga helps us take a step back and focus. Yoga calms and clears the mind, bringing us into the present moment, which in turn reduces stress and anxiety. We become more cognizant of our thoughts, words, and actions.

Boosts Confidence

Yoga makes you feel good inside and out. People of any age or body type can do yoga with some simple modifications to the poses. You may be able to extend a pose a bit longer, sit more mindfully, or notice improvement in other areas. Yoga is not something that is mastered. You are continually working and growing with it.

Promotes Health and Wellness

We practice yoga postures and breathing exercises to instill long-term benefits. Without realizing it, children are learning techniques to help make their bodies become healthier, stronger, and more relaxed as they enter their teenage and adult years. A child who learns yoga, mindfulness, and relaxation will be developing essential skills for a lifetime of health and wellness.

Chapter 2: Secrets to Teaching Yoga to Children

I love children, and I understand how to effectively teach kids yoga. I know how to engage kids, interest them in yoga, and help them learn while having fun. Although I have my adult yoga teaching certification, it would immediately heighten the stress factor for me if I were put in a room to teach adults. It's not that I don't enjoy being around adults, because I do. I just have a deep understanding of the pacing that goes into kids yoga and how to creatively interact with them.

Understanding how kids yoga differs from adult yoga can help you become more comfortable teaching yoga to children in effective and memorable ways.

1. Kids Yoga is Not Adult Yoga.

Of course you know that! Kids are obviously not adults, and they will not behave like adults. As obvious as this may seem, I really want you to take this to heart. Kids are not going to follow every pose in a structured Vinyasa adult flow class.

Most adults practice yoga to relieve tension and calm their minds, but that isn't the main goal for kids when they do yoga. They want to have fun while they learn and strengthen their bodies. Hopefully they will realize all the health benefits of yoga down the road, but right now they are just beginning.

Kids have shorter attention spans, and they like to move and interact with one another a lot. Keeping this in mind will go a long way as you introduce them to yoga.

2. Be Prepared but Flexible.

This may sound contradictory, but having a themed lesson plan in place with a breathing exercise and related yoga poses helps get the class off to an engaging start. Including a game, a read-aloud book, some group or partner work, and a moment for mindfulness and stillness will help your class have a flow and a purpose.

Be aware, though, that children are unpredictable, so be ready for anything! They have energy and varying needs and abilities. Things will happen that you didn't anticipate. Teaching yoga to kids is also about learning how to live in the moment and how to be mindful and flexible with yourself and others.

It is always good to keep in mind what you want to accomplish with the children, but being flexible allows for a greater experience for everyone.

3. Ease Up on the Alignment.

Don't take this the wrong way. Above all, be safe but not picky. Demonstrate the pose yourself and with yoga pose cards. If you spend a majority of class making sure everyone has a complete 90 degrees with their leg in Warrior 1 or that their Plank Pose includes a perfectly flat back, you will lose the attention and enthusiasm of the kids.

Yoga is a life-long journey. Our bodies are all made differently, and we are all continuing to grow and change. Our job is to introduce yoga at young ages in a way that will open the doors for a lifetime of learning, growth, and health benefits.

4. Have Fun.

Use humor. Smile. Laugh. Stay positive. Keep the mood light and somewhat spontaneous. To keep their interest and to keep them engaged, it is important to introduce the poses in a variety of ways. This is my favorite part. I enjoy creating child-friendly lesson plans that will have the kids engaged and having fun while learning. Once kids are engaged, we can then begin to implement more breathing, mindfulness, and meditation exercises so they can reap all the wonderful benefits that yoga has to offer.

Join in with the kids as well. If kids are meowing and mooing from cat pose to cow pose or dancing around the room, be sure that you are right there with them. When kids see you having fun with yoga, they will want to have fun with it as well.

5. Keep Things Moving

This secret is another favorite of mine, and one that comes easier with experience, but it is definitely one not to be missed. There is a reason that *Go Go Yoga for Kids* lesson plans include nine components. Children do not have long attention spans.

My biggest secret is to always end the games and activities on a high note, which means that everyone still wants to play. Playing a yoga game over and over and dragging it out is a sure way to have kids who "don't want to play anymore." This often means that they will start wandering around and acting up.

The recommended *Go Go Yoga for Kids* amount of time to play a game is 7-10 minutes. Always leave them wanting more. I promise that the game will be even better received the next time when you announce you are playing it.

In a children's yoga class we practice yoga postures and breathing exercises to instill lifelong benefits. Without even realizing it, children are learning techniques to help make their bodies stronger, healthier, and more mindful.

If kids are moving, trying, and having fun, they are learning. This is true for your whole class or lesson plan. Keep things moving forward, and you will have a lot fewer disruptions.

Chapter 3: Let's Get Started

Now that you know some important secrets of teaching yoga to children and understand the benefits, you are ready to get started.

Remember to feel free to adapt and pull what you need from this extended guide to make it relevant for you. If you are following the full *Go Go Yoga for Kids* lesson plans such as those given in this book, the time frame ranges from 45 minutes to one hour. If possible, I prefer to divide my classes into age appropriate groups. For example, I might separate the kids by putting 3-5 year olds together and 6-12 year olds together. However, most of these lessons and activities are applicable to both age groups.

The companion book, *Go Go Yoga for Kids: A Complete Guide to Yoga with Kids* covers in great detail every component of how to plan a kids yoga lesson. You may refer to that guide for a more in-depth look at why each component of the lesson plan is important for the whole overall flow of the class.

For those of you who are familiar with the class and lesson plan set up, here is a quick review. This plan is for a full 45-60 minute kids yoga class. If you do not have that much time, refer to the *Quick and Easy No-Time-to-Plan Kids Yoga Class* in Chapter 10 or utilize the read aloud literature books in Chapter 11. Both of these chapters provide opportunities to easily incorporate yoga with children.

Every Kids Yoga Class Includes:
1. **The Welcome:** Set the tone and theme for your class
2. **Breathing Exercises:** Focus on your breath and ways to calm your body

3. **Sun Salutations:** Practice putting your breath to movement
4. **Active Movement:** Get the wiggles out and the body warmed up
5. **Themed Yoga Poses:** Help children better retain what they have learned by using themes
6. **Yoga Games:** Practice the poses learned
7. **Partner/Group Poses or Inversion/Balance Work:** Provides an opportunity to work on those challenge poses and teamwork
8. **Community Closing:** Reflect on all that has been accomplished and learned. Share and connect together as a group one last time
9. **Stillness and Savasana:** Take time to rest, relax, and reap all the benefits of class

The following chapters will give you complete breathing exercises, poses, yoga games, favorite props to use with teaching, and mindfulness techniques to introduce to children. Feel free to add any of these into your class lesson plans.

There are also 20 ready-to-use kids yoga lesson plans in this book for your convenience. If you are unsure of any of the related yoga poses, please check the glossary for pose illustrations.

I also strongly recommend tying quality literature or read aloud books into your yoga class when it is applicable. Twelve recommended read aloud books with lesson plans are included in Chapter 12.

Finally, a blank lesson plan template is also provided to help you create your own lessons. Take what kids are interested in and notice how you are able to teach yoga to children in ways that are relevant to them. Above all, have fun introducing children to yoga.

Take what you have learned and feel confident and prepared to teach yoga to children in the school classroom, after school programs, yoga studios, summer camp, conferences, and at home with your family.

Chapter 4: Begin with Breath

Get Ready for Yoga

Breathing exercises are the best way to begin your yoga class. These exercises are also wonderful to practice at school and home. Focusing on breath helps set the tone for the rest of class and the rest of the day.

It can be difficult in the beginning to help kids learn how to slow down and become aware of their breath. Quick and shallow breaths do not make you calm and relaxed. By doing a few breathing exercises at the start of any class, children will become aware of the power of their breath, and they will begin to think of using it outside of yoga.

There are many ways to practice breathwork with kids. The following are a few favorites. Please use these and others from *Go Go Yoga for Kids: A Complete Guide to Using Yoga with Kids* to continue to introduce and use with children.

Belly Breathing

In a seated or lying down position, have the children place their hands on their stomachs. Tell each child to notice how their stomach changes as they inhale and exhale.

Birthday Candle

What child doesn't love their birthday? Kids especially love Birthday Candle Breath. Place two index fingers together as if you are holding a birthday candle. Then breathe in through your nose and breathe out your mouth as if you are blowing out a candle.

Roller Coaster Breath

Begin by holding out one hand and spreading fingers wide. This is the roller coaster and the fingers represent the hills. Use your pointer finger on the opposite hand to be the roller coaster car. Begin by pointing to your thumb and breathe out as you trace down one side of your thumb. Breathe in as you begin to trace up your pointer finger. Continue breathing in and out as you trace up and down your fingers. This is a very calming and meditative breathing exercise, unlike going on a real roller coaster.

Triangle Breath

Pretend you are drawing the shape of a triangle in front of you. Breathe in as you draw one part. Then breathe out for the other side. Finally breathe in as you connect the triangle together.

Straw Breathing

Kids love controlling their breath by practicing with a straw. Please be sure to have individual straws for the children. They can also take their straws with them to continue practicing.

Also, use a cotton ball or colored puff ball for this breathing exercise. Practice breathing slowly and steadily through the straw to make your ball move along the floor, desk, or yoga mat. What happens when you breathe quickly and fast? Notice the difference.

Snowflake Breathing

Imagine you are making it snow. Breathe in to make snowflakes fall. Breathe out and imagine snowflakes melting.

Back to Back Breath

This breathing exercise is done with a partner. Sit back to back with your partner and link arms. Take in deep breaths through your nose and then out of your mouth. Be mindful and notice your partner's breath. This exercise is especially helpful in encouraging children to take deep breaths because they want to be sure their partner will be able to feel it.

Dragon's Breath

Place your fists under your chin and inhale through your nose. Then exhale sharply with your tongue out as you move your arms down. It is almost as if you are breathing fire!

Pinwheel Breath

Pinwheels are a wonderful visual for young children to see their breath in action. Have them practice blowing the pinwheel with variations in how long or short they breathe. Notice how the pinwheel reacts. This breathing exercise can also be done with bubbles.

Breathing Buddies

It is so much fun to practice breathwork with a breathing buddy! Breathing buddies can be as simple as a little stuffed animal or plastic toy figure. I like to incorporate breathing buddies throughout a yoga class since they can be used for balance practice or an audience for our yoga show.

To practice breathwork, place a breathing buddy on your belly as you lie down. Notice the gentle rise and fall of your buddy as you breathe deeply in and out.

Breathing Ball (Hoberman Sphere)

Children enjoy this tool for breathwork exercises. Its official name is a Hoberman Sphere. Pull the sphere out as you inhale and pull it together as you exhale. This is a great visual for how your lungs or diaphragm work.

Chapter 5: How to Introduce Yoga Poses to Children

Kids love learning new yoga poses and often get excited to add new ones to their repertoire. Since kids do not have the same retention and memory as adults, I have found it helpful to group the yoga poses together by a theme. It is also helpful to only introduce three to five yoga poses per class. This really gives children the opportunity to practice the yoga poses and remember them outside of class time.

I love creating themed lesson plans with child-friendly and relevant yoga poses. I select my yoga poses from the *Kids Yoga Challenge Pose Cards*, but any other yoga pose cards would also work. It is also great when you demonstrate the pose as well, but pose cards provide a visual for the children and are helpful for practice and games.

When introducing the yoga poses, building anticipation is a great technique. I often use seasonal related items such as spring baskets, stocking caps, plastic pumpkins, sand pails, or colorful gift bags and allow the children to take turns drawing the card out.

When beginning this activity, I call on a child "with a quiet hand" to come and select our next pose. We then practice the selected pose and discuss which parts of our body we feel working and getting stronger. After we have practiced that pose, I then call on another child to draw out the next special pose. It is this simple activity that helps make it eagerly anticipated. After learning the selected yoga poses, it is then perfect timing to practice them with some yoga games.

The Top 9 Yoga Poses for Kids

The following nine yoga poses were selected for their health benefits in young growing bodies. They are wonderful for getting kids moving and active. Keep in mind that these are also adult poses, so some of them may already be familiar to you. You do not need to have a lot of space to practice these poses, and they can be done at any time to achieve the benefits. Many of them have animal names so children are able to relate to the poses.

There are additional yoga pose illustrations found in the glossary at the end of this book.

Child's Pose: Outstretch your arms and bring your forehead to the floor. Breathe deeply in and out through your nose. This is a very centering and grounding pose.

Cat Pose: Begin on your hands and knees in a table-top position. Tuck your chin and arch your back like a Halloween cat. Inhale through your nose and enjoy this stretch. On the exhale return to a neutral position.

Cow Pose: This pose pairs together very well with Cat Pose. Begin on your hands and knees in a table-top position, drop your belly, relax your spine, and look up.

It is great to practice Cat Pose to Cow Pose together since it really warms up your spine. It is especially fun with kids to practice the mooing and meowing sounds with each pose.

Updog Pose: Lie on your stomach. Place the palms of your hands next to your shoulders and look up. Slowly straighten your arms and open your chest. It is okay to keep arms bent as well. This is a wonderful pose for opening your heart.

Down Dog Pose: Begin on all fours in a table-top position. Spread your fingers and press your palms flat onto the ground.

Straighten your legs, and make an upside-down V shape. Relax your head and neck and look between your legs.

This is one of my favorite yoga poses for kids because it builds strength within your entire body. Your arms, legs, shoulders, and stomach are all working. I like to tell my students that they are getting taller as this pose lengthens their hamstrings. They love hearing this!

Boat Pose: Balance on your bottom, and lift your straightened legs in front of you. Keep a tall spine and tighten your belly. This is a good pose for building balance and strength in your core. Sometimes we row our boats and sing "Row Row Row your Boat."

Mountain Pose: Roll your shoulders back and down and stand up straight. Raise your arms and look between them. Be tall like a mountain. Kids love being big and this pose allows them to stretch up as high as they can. This pose also builds alignment, good posture, and core strength.

Ragdoll Pose: Bend over at the waist and let your arms hang like a rag doll. Gently grab the opposite elbow and sway back and forth. Feel your lower back release. This pose is great for relaxing and letting go. It is also an inversion, so children will get those upside down pose benefits, which calms the nervous system.

Tree Pose: Stand up straight and tall like in Mountain Pose. Look on the ground or find a spot that is not moving to focus on. Place your hands at heart center. Slowly bend your knee and place your foot on the inside of your other leg. Then you can raise your branches (arms) up in the air.

Chapter 6: Kids Yoga Games

Kids love yoga games. Yoga Games are a great way to get kids moving, build strength, follow directions, work together, and practice yoga poses in a fun and engaging way. Many of these games require few or no materials, but it is helpful to use yoga pose cards to provide a visual. These can be the *Kids Yoga Challenge Pose Cards* or another deck.

These games can be played with groups of any size. Yoga games that are best suited for the school classroom are indicated. For dozens of additional games, please check out *Go Go Yoga for Kids: A Complete Guide for Using Yoga with Kids*.

Downward Dog Tunnels

Materials: none

How to Play: Have the kids all line up and move into Downward Dog to create a tunnel. The child on the far end gets down on their stomach and army crawls through the tunnel. At the end, they move to Downward Dog and then the next child goes through. You can play this game as long as everyone has a turn to crawl through the tunnel. By having the kids create two separate tunnels or timing each child to see how long it takes them to get through, this game also works well as a race. They love being timed and have a lot of fun with this game.

Yoga Queen (or King)

Materials: *Kids Yoga Challenge Pose Cards*, crown (optional)

How to Play: Select someone to be the yoga queen or king. The queen or king is in command and gets to dictate to his or her subjects the yoga poses that will be performed. They call out a yoga pose and everyone must hold that pose.

The queen or king walks around, inspects everyone's pose, and crowns a new ruler.

Ring Around the Yogi

Materials: None

How to Play: This game is best suited for ages 2-5. Ring Around the Yogi is sung to the familiar tune of "Ring Around the Rosie."

Ring around the Yogi

Ring around the Yogi

Tree Pose

Tree Pose

We all fall down

Tree Pose can be substituted with a number of yoga poses, including Airplane Pose, Triangle Pose, or Cat Pose.

Yoga Bingo

Materials: Go Go Yoga for Kids Bingo Cards (available at http://www.gogoyogakids.com/bingo/), *Kids Yoga Challenge Pose Cards*, small items to mark spaces

How to Play: This is a great game to play with two or more people. Use the included Bingo cards and yoga poses (found in appendix or on web site), and make copies depending on the number of players. Place the yoga pose cards face down, and take turns picking a card. Any players who have that pose card will demonstrate the pose and mark the space on their card.

Head, Shoulders, Knees, and Toes Yoga

Materials: none

How to Play: This game can be played with a variety of ages and can be made more difficult depending on the selected pose and speed of the song.

Sing the familiar song while pointing to each of the body parts at the end of the song. At the end of the song include the yoga pose that should be demonstrated

Head, Shoulders, Knees, and Toes

Knees and Toes

Head, Shoulders, Knees and Toes

Tree Pose (other examples: Forward Fold, Triangle Pose, Dancer Pose).

Hula Hoop Tunnel

Materials: Hula Hoops

How to Play: Begin in a circle holding hands. Place a Hula Hoop in between a pair of children. They must pass the Hula Hoop around the circle by crawling through without letting go of hands. Once this is mastered, incorporate additional Hula Hoops into the circle.

Jump the Mats

Materials: A yoga mat or beach-sized towel for each child

How to Play: Place the mats in a circle. Children stand in a circle with yoga mats separating each child. The children should be standing so they are facing the person's back ahead of them. The leader gives some sort of signal by clapping their hands or beating a drum. For each beat, the children jump over the equivalent number of mats. For example, if the teacher claps twice, the children must jump over two mats. This game teaches the children to be mindful and aware of cues besides words. You can also slow down or speed up the time between jumps.

Choose Your Pose

Materials: *Kids Yoga Challenge Pose Cards*

How to Play: This is a fun game that can be played quickly when there are a few extra moments at the end of class or when transitioning from one activity to another. Choose three yoga poses for this game. The leader turns his or her back, and everyone chooses one of the three poses to hold.

The leader calls out a pose and then turns around. Everyone holding that pose wins and gets to stay in the game. Everyone else sits down. The leader again calls out a pose and then turns back around to face the group. Play continues until there is one winner.

Yoga Dice Game

Materials: Yoga Dice, *Kids Yoga Challenge Pose Cards*

How to Play: A favorite new game to play is the Yoga Dice Game. For this game you need large a inflatable dice. Select six different poses from the *Kids Yoga Challenge Pose Cards*. Use clear tape to attach the poses to different sides of the dice. Each player takes a turn to roll the dice. The players do whatever pose is rolled. The player that makes that pose first gets to roll the dice next. Continue rolling the dice until all of the poses are mastered.

Rock/Tree/Bridge Relay

Materials: None

How to Play: This game works well with groups of three. The first child becomes a rock by getting into child's pose. The second child jumps over the "rock" and becomes a "tree." The third child jumps over the "rock," goes around the "tree," and becomes a "bridge" in Down Dog pose. The first child, who was the rock, goes around the tree and underneath the bridge. The children repeat this pattern until one team reaches the end.

Yoga Show

Materials: *Kids Yoga Challenge Pose Cards*

How to Play: Give each pair of children or small group a beginning and an ending yoga pose. They can create whatever flow, dance, or movement they want in between these two yoga poses. They can then show off their Yoga Show to the rest of the class.

This game works well with school-aged kids as well as tween or teen-aged classes. They love putting together their own flows.

Musical Mats

Materials: yoga mats, music, yoga pose cards

How to Play: Musical Mats is similar to Musical Chairs and is a way to practice many different poses. Place all of the yoga mats in a circle with a different pose card at the top of each mat.

Play music and allow the children to move in a circle around the mats. When the music stops, the children must choose a mat and hold the pose that is found at the top of the mat. Continue to play again. Depending on the ages of the children, I sometimes remove a mat and pose card each time, ultimately declaring a winner or two. For younger ages, I do not recommend anyone getting "out," but the older children sometimes enjoy a little friendly competition.

Invent a Pose

Materials: bag of stuffed or plastic animals

Begin with a bag of stuffed or plastic animals. Each child takes a turn drawing an animal out of the bag. Think of a pose that would resemble the animal. Be the teacher and teach that pose to the rest of the class.

Toega

Materials: colored pom-pom balls

How to Play: Scatter the pom-pom balls on the ground. Have the children try to pick up the colored balls with their toes and then place the balls on their yoga mat or another flat surface. To change up the game create different challenges by having the older children collect balls of the same color or size. You can also implement a time limit to see how many they can gather in one minute with their toes.

After the children have gathered their pom-pom balls, bring a connection or close to the activity by having the children sort them in groups. Leave it open ended and see what they come up with. They will often sort the balls by size and color, but once in a while I get an unexpected response, and that is lots of fun.

I Love Yoga and This is My Pose

Materials: none

How to Play: Have the children stand in a circle. One child begins by saying, "I love yoga, and this is my pose." The child then makes the pose and says the name of the pose. Then the whole group makes that pose. The next person in line does the same thing, but after doing their pose, the whole group must remember and do the first pose before doing the new one. The game continues in a circle with more and more poses being added.

Yoga Twister

Materials: Twister mat and spinner

How to Play: Begin with a normal game of Twister. After a few spins, the leader calls out, "Twister freeze!" The children playing must "freeze" and then come up with a name for a yoga pose they are holding. These can be real poses or made up. This is a fun way for kids to be creative with yoga poses and to practice flexibility.

You can add a twist on this game for older children by allowing them to come up with a name for the pose the entire group is holding as a collective. What shape does everyone all together make as opposed to a single pose and person?

Yoga Pictures

Materials: Marker board (or large paper), *Kids Yoga Challenge Pose Cards*

How to Play: Play this with teams of two or more members. Both teams choose one member to be the "drawer." Every drawer selects the same pose card. They then draw the pose the best that they can. Stick figures are fine. Each team tries to guess the name of the pose being drawn. When guessed correctly everyone on that team demonstrates it.

Ball Pass

Materials: beach ball or any type of ball

How to Play: This game works well in a tight circle. Any type of ball will work. First, tell the children to pass the ball around the circle with their hands. This allows everyone to touch the ball, which is usually what children, especially younger ages, cannot wait to do. After touching the ball, they are then better able to focus on the rest of the game.

Pass the ball around once for practice and then time it. Tell the children to focus on passing the ball to the person next to them. After passing with hands, tell the children to pass the ball using their feet. Kids are usually excited about trying to master this. This exercise requires a lot of core strength and teamwork. See if they can get faster by going the opposite direction.

Plow Race

Materials: Ball

How to Play: Plow Race is another type of ball pass game and works well with older children. Have the children sit up tall with their legs in front of them in a line. They should be facing the person's back in front of them. The child at the front of the line begins with a ball between their feet. He or she rolls to Plow Pose on their back to pass the ball to the person sitting behind them. That person grabs the ball with their feet and repeats. This game is also fun to use as a relay or a race.

School Based Yoga Games

The following games can be played during a kids yoga class, but they also work well in the school classroom. They do not need a lot of materials, and large groups can enjoy playing them.

Noisy Bell/Quiet Bell

Materials: small bell

How to Play: This game is absolutely a favorite of kids and is perfect for working on patience and mindfulness. Sit in a circle and pass the bell around to show how noisy it can be. Then challenge the children to pass the bell as quietly as possible.

You can also have the students get up and pass the bell to someone across the room without making a sound. They are completely mesmerized by this.

Pick a Card

Materials: *Kids Yoga Challenge Pose Cards*

How to Play: Fan the *Kids Yoga Challenge Pose Cards* out and allow the child who is first to get to the carpet after center time or transitions to select a card. Everyone holds that pose while waiting for the next class directions. Since they are actively doing something, this game is a better option than just having the kids sit and wait for everyone to be ready.

Instinct

Materials: A small object

How to Play: This quiet game is perfect for winding down after a busy class. It allows the children to practice being aware and mindful and teaches them to pay attention to their intuition. Tell the children to sit quietly on mats that have been placed in a circle. If you do not have yoga mats, just have the children sit in a circle.

One child leaves the room or goes to a corner and turns his or her back on the class. Another child hides the object somewhere in the mat circle. The first child comes back into the room and is given three guesses to use his or her instinct to find where the object is hidden.

Pose of the Week

Materials: *Kids Yoga Challenge Pose Cards*

How to Play: Post the pose of the week, such as Tree Pose or Mountain Pose, in a designated spot in the classroom. When the Pose of the Week is called, everyone stops what they are doing and makes that pose. This is a great exercise because students will respond better to this active pose than telling everyone to be quiet. Students are not only listening, but they are also getting some stretching and movement in.

Count while holding a Balance Pose

Materials: Select balance poses from the *Kids Yoga Challenge Pose Cards* such as Tree Pose, Dancer Pose, Airplane Pose, One Legged Mountain Pose, etc.

How to Play: This is a great game to work on balance as well as school skills. Practice counting by two's, five's, 10's, or other multiples. This game also works well while standing in line waiting for everyone. Try even counting in Spanish or backwards to keep it fresh.

Chapter 7: Top 12 Props to Use in Teaching Kids Yoga

Having a few props on hand while teaching yoga to children can help keep them active and engaged. Over the years, I have tried and tested dozen of items to use in my kids yoga classes to find out which ones work well for teaching and are fun for the kids.

There is no need to spend a lot of money on yoga props. Most of these items are inexpensive and might even be found in your own home. Do not feel the need to use these props all at once. It is best to bring them out for a short while and then tuck them away to help keep the anticipation and interest level high. I always carry a few in my yoga bag and rotate them out.

1. Feathers

There are many uses for feathers in yoga. Feathers are great tools when doing breathing exercises with kids. Give each child a feather and tell them to control their breathing by blowing the feather up and down their yoga mat. Feathers can also be used in pairs or a group. Another option is to line the children up at one end of the room. Have them keep track of their feather as they blow it across the room on their hands and knees.

2. Pom-Pom Balls

These inexpensive colored balls are also wonderful to use during breathing exercises and for teaching children the importance of taking big, deep breaths. Use them as tools for games similar to what you would do with feathers. They can also be used to play the very popular Toega Yoga Game.

3. Beanbags

Beanbags are fabulous to use for balance work. Children can try to hold balance poses such as Tree Pose or Dancer Pose while balancing beanbags on their heads. It is also fun to use beanbags as a walking balance challenge. Have the children line up on one end of the room. They can practice holding the beanbag on their elbow, under their chin, or on top of their head as they slowly walk across the room. Begin with the easier balance exercises first such as holding it under the chin and work up to the more challenging ones. Remind the children that this is not a race. They are working on staying focused and mindful and not letting their beanbag drop.

Beanbags can also be used as "Breathing Buddies" for when children are slowing down and being mindful of their breath. I like to have the children lie down and notice the beanbag moving up and down with their deep breathing.

4. Yoga Pose Cards

It is extremely beneficial to have visuals for children as they are learning and practicing yoga. There are a variety of yoga pose cards available and many have certain strong points.

One of my favorites of these is the *Kids Yoga Challenge Pose Cards,* which were created with a teacher in mind. The 40 progressive yoga poses are unique in that they are leveled by difficulty. Children try to master Level 1 before moving on to Level 2 and so forth. These cards also include partner poses which children absolutely love. There are also many games that can be played with yoga pose cards.

5. Hoberman Sphere (Breathing Ball)

This engaging toy is perfect for leading breathing exercises with children. This breathing ball mimics the diaphragm and shows the importance of taking deep breaths and expanding your lungs.

As you stretch the ball out, take a long deep breath together as a group. Then as you squeeze the ball together, let out a long deep exhale. You can experiment with the pace and show what happens when we breathe in and out too quickly. Talk about the difference in how your body feels when you take short, quick breaths compared to long, deep breaths.

If you are working with a smaller group, pass the ball around the circle and let each child take turns opening and closing it in time with their breath.

The ball is also fun to toss around the circle as it opens and shuts. Have the children participate in a team building and cooperation exercise to see how many times they can catch the ball without it dropping. This is also a good exercise in building mindfulness. These balls can be purchased in different sizes. The one that I use the most is the "mini" and works just fine with children.

6. Literature Books (Read Alouds)

This is a favorite! Sharing a good quality book with children can definitely enhance a yoga experience for kids. It is also wonderful to tie together an overlying theme or message. See Read Aloud Books Chapter 12.

7. Balls

All different shapes and sizes of balls work well. Balls can be used in ball-pass games and as a prop for taking turns in the Community Building portion of class. Children enjoy using balls for seated ball back massages on one another, and they can be rolled down children's backs while they are holding Plank Pose. The uses are endless, and I always have a few on hand anytime I am teaching yoga to children.

8. Hula Hoops

This inexpensive prop is perfect for many yoga games and activities. I love to use hoops to create a yoga obstacle course for children to jump between. They are perfect for cooperative game activities such as holding hands and trying to pass the hoop around the circle. I also use them as a stage for a child to showcase a certain balance pose such as Tree Pose or Airplane Pose since those poses work well within perimeters of the hoop.

9. Focal Points

Focal points can be small objects such as a stuffed animal, gemstone, sticker, or anything of interest that you have on hand. I always remind my students to look at the floor while they are holding their balance poses. I have found that by focusing on a stationary object, children are better able to focus and therefore hold their balance in poses.

10. Dry Erase Board and Marker

Dry Erase Boards have so many uses. Any size works well. They can be used for games such as Yoga Pictures (see Yoga Games Chapter 6). I also really like to draw a shape on them such as a circle or triangle and then challenge the children to make that shape with their body. They can also work in pairs or small groups to make shapes that are shown on the dry erase board. If working in small groups, challenge the children by seeing if they can make the shape or letter silently while working together.

11. Jump Ropes

I always carry a couple of jump ropes with me to a kids yoga class. These are wonderful for using in a yoga obstacle course for "jumping a river." These jump ropes can be laid side by side so the area between them is the "river." Kids love trying to jump across the river and not fall in.

I also like to use jump ropes for a rope walk game which is perfect for meditation and focus. While barefoot, children try to stay on the line while walking slowly with foot to heel. It is harder than it appears, and children really need to slow down and focus in order to complete the challenge.

12. Seasonal Related Items

I love to introduce our yoga poses with a seasonal item. For example, poses could be written on slips of paper and placed in Easter eggs. Children then take turns drawing an egg and discovering the next pose to learn. They could also draw poses out of plastic pumpkins, gift bags, sand pails, present boxes, etc. Kids will absolutely be drawn right in when you pull out your seasonal item. I also like to pair the poses with the themed lesson plans. See Chapter 9 for kids yoga lesson plans.

Chapter 8: Building Mindfulness in Children Through Moving Meditation and Mantras

When I use yoga with kids, the energy level varies. I like to begin at a low level, focusing on our breath and being calm and mindful. Then I move into yoga poses and games, which require a mid- to high-energy level. Finally, I like to bring the level back down with relaxation. Kids do really well with this type of pacing in a yoga class.

Throughout our time together I consistently try to model mindfulness in ourselves and with others. We begin with being mindful of our breath, then being mindful of how our bodies feel holding the yoga poses, and finally being mindful of one another during our partner poses or group challenges.

Of course, mindfulness can be taught other places besides in a yoga class. The following exercises would work well at home, school, or a studio.

All of the breathing exercises in Chapter Four work well for building mindfulness, but I have also included other activities that help build awareness in children.

Moving Meditation and Mantras

One way to build mindfulness is through a moving meditation or mantra. Mantras are similar to affirmations, and over time they can help change the way we feel. Mantras are repeated over and over to ourselves out loud or silently. It is a wonderful technique for kids to use to set themselves up for doing their best and feeling good about themselves and their efforts.

When developing the *Kids Yoga Challenge Pose Cards*, mantras and affirmations were absolutely something that I wanted to include. Yoga poses make you feel good, and when you combine that with the included affirmations, it empowers the children even more.

Each of the yoga pose cards includes a pose with a relevant mantra. By selecting poses, practicing them and repeating the mantra, you have children who are receiving both mental and physical benefits.

Do not worry if you do not have the *Kids Yoga Challenge Pose Cards*. You can still include mantras with the yoga poses that you introduce. Just ask the kids. They are sure to have good ideas on how the poses make them feel.

As children progress in yoga, it is powerful to include a moving meditation with their yoga practice. This includes several poses and related mantras.

The following mantra is one of my favorites that I use often with my kids yoga classes. I like to flow through it a couple of times at the beginning of class. What I like about it is that the kids are moving while saying the mantra. This helps provide greater understanding and meaning as they hold the yoga pose and feel empowered.

We repeat the following mantra as part of our Sun Salutation warm up at the beginning of class.

Go Go Yoga for Kids Mantra

Hands at Heart Center: I am Calm

Warrior 1: I am Confident

Warrior 2: I am Strong

Reverse Warrior: I am Mindful

Hands at Heart Center: I am Ready

The following ideas are favorites of mine to also incorporate mindfulness in children. Once learned, they will be able to practice these on their own.

Body Scan

This simple mindfulness exercise helps kids calm down and relax. The body scan is also a fun exercise for building awareness of how emotions impact our bodies. Emotions are not just experienced in our minds, but they are also felt in the body. Think about that sinking feeling you get in your stomach or the weight of stress on the shoulders.

As adults we tend to hold stress up in our shoulders, but kids often hold their emotions in their gut. This makes sense for those of you who work closely with children. Many times there are tummy aches, and they aren't necessarily always from being sick or hungry.

The more we pay attention to how our body feels, the more we can pay attention to subtle clues and adjust accordingly. In other words, don't let a bad mood escalate into more.

How to do a Body Scan:

This activity gets the children to think about parts of their body that they often don't pay attention to. Some of it may seem silly to little ones at first, so model it aloud first, and be sure to state what you are feeling and how you are relaxing your body parts.

1. Allow the children to lie down in a comfortable position and close their eyes.
2. Have them observe their breath and notice the natural inhales and exhales.
3. Move their attention to the top of their head, including their scalp and hair.

4. Next include the back of the head, forehead, and eyes, including eyelashes and eyebrows.
5. Continue to move their attention throughout their bodies, working from the top down. Pause at each area to see if they can relax it even more. When that area feels completely relaxed, move on to the next area.
6. At the end, tell them to connect their whole body together as they feel breath moving throughout their bodies.
7. Continue to breathe and relax as long as they need.

A good tip is to provide a visual for children. You can do this by helping them focus on tense or sore areas in their bodies. Help them to imagine that those sore areas are fire and their breath is like ice. Focus in on that area until it is relaxed and cool.

Another visualization technique is to tell the children to imagine a magic wand gently sweeping over each area and calming and relaxing them.

Finally, another idea for a body scan that has worked well with children and adults is for them to squeeze and relax each area as they move through their body. This effort sometimes helps with pinpointing exactly what area they are focusing on.

Make a Mindfulness Jar

Making a mindfulness jar is a simple thing to do, but it provides a wonderful visual for children and adults on the importance of managing our emotions.

How to make a Mindfulness Jar

What you need:

Clear jar (such as a mason jar)

Glitter (one to three colors)

A few drops of clear soap

Fill the jar to the top with water and add a few drops of dish soap. Drop a few pinches of glitter into the jar. Close or seal the jar tightly.

How to use a Mindfulness Jar:

The jar is like our mind. Each speck of glitter focuses on different thoughts. Focus on the glitter specks and imagine each one as a stressor or worry (school, test, family). Shake up the jar and see how all of the stressors swirl around your mind. What can you do to slow things down and help your mind become clear again?

Be still. Breathe. Over time everything will settle down. Our thoughts are still there, but they have settled and calmed.

I also like to use Mindfulness Jars as a drishti or focal point for balance work. I often remind children to look at a spot on the floor that is not moving to help them stay balanced. By placing a Mindfulness Jar in the room, it provides something that all of the children want to look at while practicing Tree Pose, Airplane Pose, or Dancer Pose.

Additionally, all of the breathing exercises in Chapter 4 work well for building mindfulness. *Go Go Yoga for Kids: A*

Complete Guide to Yoga with Kids includes many additional ideas on building mindfulness in children.

Chapter 9: Introduction to Kids Yoga Lesson Planning

Having a lesson plan or guide in place will help you be prepared for teaching yoga to kids. That doesn't mean you can't be in the moment and flexible, but it does help you be prepared. The attention span of children is short, much shorter than adults. It is important to have a variety of props and activities to help your class run smoothly and accomplish what you want with the time that you have.

Go Go Yoga for Kids: A Complete Guide to Using Yoga with Kids covers in full detail each component of teaching a kids yoga class and why each part is important. This follow-up guide assumes that you are comfortable with each of the components needed to put together an effective kids yoga class.

There are three different templates available in this resource to help you with your lesson planning. Each one offers a different visual appeal so pick and choose as to what works best for you.

Each lesson plan is theme related based on kids' interests and skills. It has been demonstrated that children will remember the poses and lesson better if it follows a sequence and a theme.

The lesson plans are based on a 45-60 minute kids yoga class. That doesn't mean you need to use every part or component. Pick and choose whatever works best for you and the needs of your class.

Enjoy and have fun teaching yoga to children!

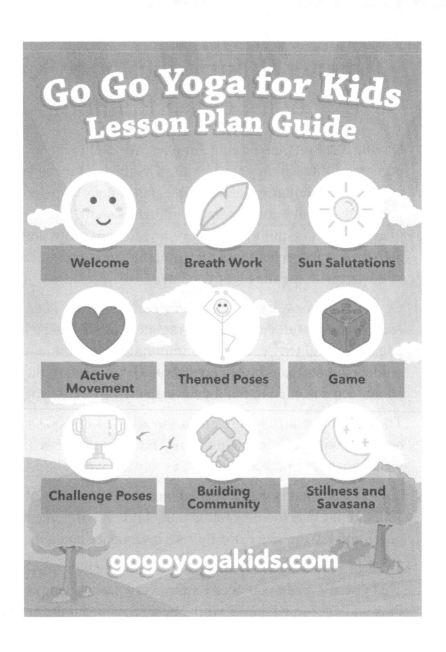

Go Go Yoga for Kids

Lesson Plan Template

Theme:	
Ages:	
Materials:	
Welcome:	
Breath Work:	
Sun Salutation:	
Active Movement:	
Theme Poses:	
Yoga Game:	
Partner/Group Challenge Poses: OR Inversion/Balance:	
Community Closing:	

Go Go Yoga for Kids

Lesson Plan

Theme

Materials

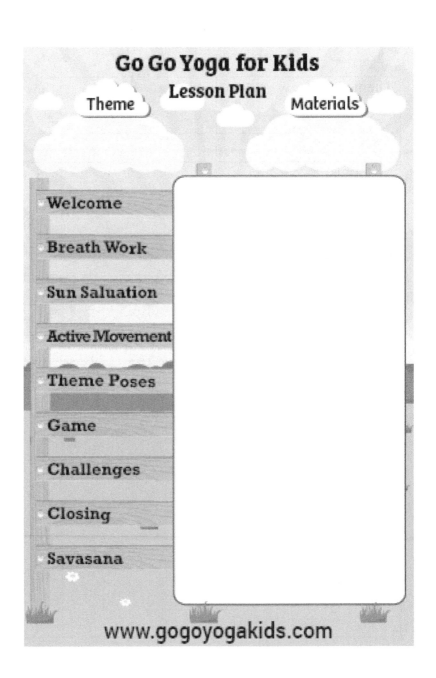

- Welcome
- Breath Work
- Sun Saluation
- Active Movement
- Theme Poses
- Game
- Challenges
- Closing
- Savasana

www.gogoyogakids.com

Page 50

Chapter 10: Lesson Plans

Theme:	A Trip to the Farm
Ages:	2-5
Materials:	Music
Welcome:	What kinds of animals do you see on the farm?
Breath Work:	**Animal Breath:** Pick an animal that lives on a farm such as a cow, sheep, or horse. Take a deep breath and on the exhale make the animal sound.
Sun Salutation:	**Sun A:** Rise and shine and act as a rooster waking up the barnyard.
Active Movement:	**Barnyard Dance:** Begin by designating each corner of the room as the farm animal's pen. Allow the children to choose which pen or corner they want to go in. When the farmer shouts, "Barnyard dance!" all of the animals come out of their pens to the center of the room to dance and move. When the farmer says, "Time for bed," all of the animals must move back to their pen.

Theme Poses:	**Cow Pose to Cat Pose:** Make the animal sound as you transition between the poses.
	Horse Pose: Can you neigh like a horse?
	Chicken (Duck Pose): Flap your wings and move your head back and forth.
	Farm Dog: (Down Dog Pose)
Game:	**Farmer in the Dell:** Join hands and move in a circle as you sing or play this childhood favorite song. Select different children to be the animals in the center of the circle.
Community Closing:	**Animal Showcase:** Have each child take a turn demonstrating their favorite animal pose that they learned. They can also make up their own.
Stillness and Savasana:	Time for all of the barnyard animals to take a rest in their pen.

Theme:	African Safari Adventure
Ages:	3-11
Materials:	None
Welcome:	What do you know about Africa?
Breath Work:	**Lion's Breath:** Take a deep inhale through your nose, then open your mouth wide, stick your tongue out, and exhale with a distinct "Ha" sound.
Sun Salutation:	**Mount Kilimanjaro to the Nile River:** Breathe in and begin in Mountain Pose with arms overhead. Exhale and dive forward with arms outstretched as if diving into the Nile River. Repeat several times.
Active Movement:	**Animal Walks:** Move slowly like an elephant, fast like a tiger, and slither like a snake.
Theme Poses:	**Lion** (Cat Pose): Arch your back and roar.

	Giraffe (Tree Pose): Reach both arms up as if you are a giraffe trying to reach the tall leaves. **Elephant:** In a one arm Down Dog, sway your arm as if it is an elephant's trunk. **Cobra** (Updog Pose): Lift your head and belly off the ground and hiss like a snake.
Game:	**Sleeping Safari Animals:** All of the children except for one or two hunters freeze in a safari animal yoga pose. The hunters walk around the room and try to wake up the sleeping animals by being silly or telling jokes. They are not allowed to touch the animals. If one of the "animals" moves, then he or she becomes the next hunter.
Partner/Group Challenge Poses:	**Double Cobra Partner Pose:** Each pair goes into Cobra Pose facing one another. They then lift

	their heads and connect their arms at the top.
Community Closing:	**Share Good Moments**: While sitting in a circle, have each child take a turn sharing one or two good or positive moments from the class.
Stillness and Savasana:	**Silent Safari Savasana:** See who can be the quietest animal in the Safari for a few moments.

Theme:	Australian Adventure
Ages:	3-11
Materials:	None
Welcome:	What do you know about Australia? What animals are from there? What are some places to visit?
Breath Work:	**Didgeridoo Breath**: A didgeridoo is a wind instrument made from hollow wood. Pretend to hold this long instrument in your hands. Breathe in and breathe out deeply to fill this instrument with air.
Sun Salutation:	Sun A
Active Movement:	Australia is a long ways away, and we will need an airplane to get there. Stand on one leg in Airplane Pose and balance as long as you are able. Then switch legs and balance so they will both be equal.
Theme Poses:	**Koala** (Eagle Pose): Pretend you are a Koala wrapping yourself around a tree branch.

	Kangaroo (Chair Pose): Bend knees and hop forward like a kangaroo.
	Platypus (Bow Pose): Pretend to glide through the water on your belly.
	Jellyfish (Ragdoll Pose): Gently sway from side to side.
Game:	**Great Barrier Reef:** The Great Barrier Reef is the world's largest coral reef system. Begin with half of the children forming part of the reef by choosing a yoga pose to hold and become the coral. These children must each be touching one another and be connected in some way. The remaining children become fish and must pass through the reef without touching part of the coral. If the fish touch the coral while passing through then they become part of the coral reef. Play continues until there are one or two

	fish left. Begin again with a new coral reef structure.
Partner/Group Challenge Poses: OR Inversion/Balance:	**Down Dog Tunnel:** Drive through the Sydney Harbor Bridge with this group yoga pose. Everyone goes into Down Dog pose close to one another. Take turns crawling through the tunnel.
Community Closing:	**Pass the Squeeze:** Children sit up tall in a circle while holding hands. The first person squeezes the person's hand next to them. Let the squeeze continue around the circle until it works its way back to the one who started it.
Stillness and Savasana:	Be like a koala and do what koalas do best...sleep.

Theme:	**Circus Yoga**
Ages:	3-7
Materials:	Jump rope or masking tape
Welcome:	What kinds of things do you see at the circus?
Breath Work:	**Lion's Breath**: Kneel with your bottom resting on your heels. Inhale through your nose. Exhale strongly through your mouth, making a "ha" sound. As you exhale, open your mouth wide and stick your tongue as far out as possible.
Sun Salutation:	Sun A
Active Movement:	Pretend to ride your unicycle in the circus (bicycle crunches).
Theme Poses:	**Seal** (Updog Pose): Can you clap your hands as if you are a seal in the circus? **Elephant:** In a one arm Down Dog, sway your arm as if it is a trunk.

	Tight Rope Walker: (Dancer Pose) **Performer:** (Star Pose)
Game:	**Walk the Tightrope:** Put the jump ropes down or make a path with masking tape across the floor. The tightrope walkers need to mindfully walk along the rope. Encourage them to step carefully heel to toe so they do not fall off.
Partner/Group Challenge Poses:	**Circus Tent:** Make a circus tent with your partner with this fun partner pose. Stand facing one another with palms touching overhead. Each partner takes a small step back while keeping the palms touching. Raise your arms up together to form a tent.
Community Closing:	**Circus Show:** Everyone takes a moment to think of their favorite pose or circus act. Each person then takes a moment to show their "act" in the center of the circle.

Stillness and Savasana:	The circus is over. It is time to rest and relax.

Theme:	Birthday Yoga
Ages:	3-10
Welcome:	What do you like about your birthday?
Breath Work:	**Candle Breath:** Put your index fingers together as if they are a candle. Breathe in. As you exhale, try to blow out your candle.
	Balloon Breath: Sit comfortably and breathe. On the inhale, bring your arms overhead to make a balloon shape with your fingertips. On the exhale, let the air out of your balloon by bringing your palms together and back to heart center.
Sun Salutation:	**Sun A:** Show how much you have grown this year by inhaling and stretching your arms up high overhead, then dive forward as you exhale.
Active Movement:	**Make a Yoga Birthday Cake**: Sit up tall and put the heels of your feet together to create a bowl to mix your cake. Ask the

	children which ingredients are needed to make the cake. Reach your arms up high for each ingredient (eggs, butter, flour, and sugar). Then bring them down low into the bowl. Use your arms to stir the batter. Put the cake into the oven by closing your knees. Pretend to set the timer and tick tock back and forth. When the timer goes off, frost the cake with big sweeping motions with your arms and then enjoy.
Theme Poses:	**Candle** (Shoulder Stand Pose): Bring your hands to your lower back and lift into a candlestick or Shoulder Stand with your toes pointed.
	Table (Reverse Plank Pose): Sit on the floor and plant your hands behind you, fingers facing forward. Plant your feet firmly and lift your bottom toward the ceiling.

	Chair Pose: Set your bottom back down as if you are sitting in a chair. **Star Pose:** You are the birthday star. Enjoy!
Game:	**Happy Birthday:** Everyone is seated in a circle and goes into Shoulder Stand Pose while singing "Happy Birthday." The birthday child will walk around the circle to blow out each of the candles. When the song ends, whoever is nearest at the end of the song becomes the next birthday child.
Partner/Group Challenge Poses:	**Group Table and Chairs:** Everyone sits in a line and comes into table pose so it looks like a long dining room table in which to enjoy your birthday cake. Some kids can volunteer to be the chairs next to the table.
Community Closing:	**Pretend Presents**: Take turns pretending to give a present to each child. Mix it up by acting as if some

	are heavy or unusually shaped. Each child takes a moment to "unwrap" his present and show how he would use it. Everyone can take turns guessing.
Stillness and Savasana:	Lie down slowly as if you are a balloon losing air. Be comfortable on your back, side, or stomach.

Theme:	**Surf's Up: Hawaii Yoga**
Ages:	3-11
Materials:	Music
Welcome:	What do you know about surfing or Hawaii? Have you ever seen someone surfing or tried it yourself?
Breath Work:	**Ocean Breath:** Seal your lips and begin to breathe in and out through your nose. The inhales are similar to the sound an ocean makes as water is gathering up to form the wave. The exhales can be compared to the sound of the waves crashing to the shore. This is also called Ujjayi breath.
Sun Salutation:	**Ocean Dive Sun A:** Now take that same Ocean Breath and add movement. Breathe in and stretch your arms up overhead. Breathe out and dive forward over your knees.
Active Movement:	**Surfer Jumps:** Begin in Warrior 2 position. Then jump and switch lead legs. Be sure to get some "hang time" on your jumps.
Theme Poses:	**Surfer:** (Warrior 2)

	Palm Tree: (Tree Pose)
	Shark (Bow Pose): Lie on your belly. Place your hands on your back as if they are the fins of a shark. Lift your head and legs.
	Swimmer: Lie on your belly and move your arms and legs as if swimming
Game:	**Surf Board Scramble:** Place yoga mats in a circle. Play music and everyone moves or dances while moving in a circle. When the music stops, everyone must find a yoga mat surfboard and hold a pose that they have just learned.
Partner/Group Challenge Poses:	**Group Tree Challenge:** Surfers need to have good balance. Everyone stands close together in a circle and holds hands with the person next to them. Next they move into Tree Pose. Have everyone raise their arms up. Try closing one eye and then both to test your balance.
Community Closing:	**Surf Board Yoga:** Children sit in a circle. Next place a yoga mat in the center to be the surfboard. Each "surfer" takes a

	moment to go in the center of the circle and demonstrate a yoga pose as if they are on a surfboard or paddle board.
Stillness and Savasana:	Even surfers need to rest. Lie down as still as possible on your surf board.

Theme:	**Jump into Fall**
Ages:	3-11
Materials:	None
Welcome:	What do you love about the fall season? (Examples: pumpkins, apples, trick or treating).
Breath Work:	Children breathe in and out deeply as if taking in the crisp fall air.
Sun Salutation:	**Sun A**
Active Movement:	**Pumpkin Rolls:** Students hug their knees in tight and roll up and down on their mat.
Theme Poses:	**Leaf:** (Star Pose) **Apple Basket:** (Boat Pose) **Bat**: (Airplane Pose) **Pumpkin:** (Child's Pose) **Scarecrow:** (Tree Pose)
Game:	**Wind Through the Trees:** Half of the children stand in tree pose near one another as if they are a forest. The other half of the students move in and out of the trees as if they are the wind. The "wind" is not allowed to touch the "trees." The trees need to try to keep their balance.

Partner/Group Challenge Poses:	**Bat Cave:** The students make a Down Dog Tunnel. One student needs to crawl through the tunnel as if he or she is a bat. Each student takes a turn as the bat.
Community Closing:	**Circle Showcase:** Everyone takes a moment and shows a favorite pose they have learned.
Stillness and Savasana:	Children sit up tall with legs out in front. Have them lay back very slowly onto their backs as if they are a leaf falling to the ground.

Theme:	**Let's Be Thankful:** Learn about gratitude and being thankful all year long.
Ages:	3-11
Materials:	One rock
Welcome:	What are you thankful for?
Breath Work:	**Turkey Breath:** Sit cross-legged and make turkey feathers by breathing in and outstretching your arms up overhead. Clasp your hands at the top and bring them to heart center with a "gobble, gobble, gobble."
Sun Salutation:	**Sun A:** Give thanks for the sun as you reach your arms up overhead and dive forward.
Active Movement:	**Turkey Trot:** How would a turkey move? Move around the room and get the wiggles out before learning our thankful themed poses.
Theme Poses:	We are thankful for all of these things on our earth. **Mountains** (Mountain Pose): Reach your arms

	overhead and look between your hands. **Flowers** (Lotus Pose): Sit cross-legged and make petals with your arms overhead. **Birds:** (Airplane Pose) **Trees** (Tree Pose): Bring your hands to heart center or stretch your arms up toward the sky. **Moon:** (Half Moon Pose) **Stars:** (Star Pose)
Game:	**Planksgiving:** Make a Thanksgiving table together as a group. Demonstrate **Plank Pose**. Have all of the children practice the pose. Next have the students practice **Chair Pose**. Bring it all together by having the children take turns being the table and chairs for the perfect Thanksgiving feast.
Community Closing:	**Gratitude Rock:** We have so many things to be thankful for. Take turns passing the gratitude rock around the circle with

	everyone taking a turn saying what they are thankful for.
Stillness and Savasana:	Have the children lie on their backs while hugging their knees in tight and giving themselves a hug. Then have them lie still and slowly squeeze and relax each body part beginning with their toes and moving up their legs, hands, and eyes until finally relaxing into their final resting pose.

Theme:	**Let's Eat: A Yoga Adventure**
Ages:	3-10
Materials:	None
Welcome:	What are some of your favorite foods?
Breath Work:	**Cool off the Cocoa Breath:** Pretend as if you are holding a cup of hot cocoa. Use deep inhales and exhales to cool off your cocoa.
Sun Salutation:	**Apple Picking Sun A:** Pretend to be picking apples at the top of a high tree. Inhale and reach up to get the apple and on the exhale dive forward to place your apple in the basket. Repeat several times.
Active Movement:	**Egg Rolls**: Hug your knees and rock forward and back. **Pop Popcorn:** Squat down low and jump up as high as you can as if

	you are a kernel of popcorn popping. **Yoga Sandwich:** Sit with your legs outstretched in front of you. They are one slice of bread. Ask the children what they would like on their sandwich. Reach up high and pretend to get the "lettuce, pickles, peanut butter, etc.," and then bring it down low to spread it on your legs. After your sandwich is all built, fold your body over your legs to create the top of the sandwich.
Theme Poses:	Get the table set for dinner with these poses. **Table:** Reverse Plank **Bowl:** Boat Pose **Chair:** Chair Pose **Candle Stick:** Shoulder Stand Pose
Game:	**Create a Pose:** Have the children think of a food and pose that could look

	like that food and let everyone guess. For example, Triangle Pose could be a pizza slice, Lotus Pose could become a pretzel, or Shoulder Stand could be a banana. Let them be creative with moving their bodies. It does not need to be an actual yoga pose.
Inversion/Balance:	**Create a High Top Table** (L-Dog Inversion): Get into Down Dog Pose with your heels against a wall. Slowly climb your feet up the wall until your legs are level with your hips, which shapes the letter "L." This is a great exercise for building upper body strength and builds confidence as well.
Community Closing:	**Spaghetti Test:** Allow the children to relax on their backs. Perform the "Spaghetti Test" to see how relaxed they are by picking up their legs one

	at a time and gently releasing.
Stillness and Savasana:	**Make a Yoga Burrito**: Have each child lie at one end of their yoga mat with arms at their side. Next, gently roll them up with the yoga mat. This creates a nice safe place for a quiet Savasana.

Theme:	**Let's Go Camping**
Ages:	3-10
Welcome:	Who has gone camping before? What did you do? What did you see?
Breath Work:	**S'more Breath:** Sit up straight and pretend to cool off your toasted marshmallow with your deep breath. Breathe in through your nose and exhale slowly through your open mouth.
Sun Salutation:	Sun A
Active Movement:	**Going on a Bear Hunt:** This familiar song is perfect for kids to pretend to hike and a great way to add movement.
Theme Poses:	**Tent:** (Down Dog Pose) **Canoe:** (Boat Pose) **Fire:** (Firelog Pose) **Compass:** (Triangle Pose) **Moon:** (Half Moon Pose)
Game:	**Bears in the Forest:** This yoga game is perfect for active movement and balance work. Half of the kids work on tree pose while the other children bear walk through the trees. See if the "trees" can keep their

	focus while the bears walk between them.
Partner/Group Challenge Poses	**Create a Campground:** Children form a Down Dog Tunnel to look like a row of tents. They can also add a fire, canoe, or any other pose they have learned.
Community Closing:	**Fire Pit:** Turn the lights off. Everyone rolls up their yoga mat into a log shape. Take turns adding a log to the fire. Everyone can sit around the "fire" and share a favorite part of class.
Stillness and Savasana:	The moon and stars are out, and it is time for stillness. Lie down quietly on your yoga mat sleeping bag. You deserve this yoga break after all of your adventures.

Theme:	**Share the Love Yoga**
Ages:	5-12
Materials:	None
Welcome:	What are some ways you can show someone that you love them?
Breath Work:	**Share the Love:** Breathe in deeply to take in love as you raise your arms up overhead. Then exhale strongly to share the love as you bring your hands back to heart center.
Sun Salutation:	**Sun A:** Begin standing with hands at heart center. On the inhale, raise your arms above your head. On the exhale, dive forward over your legs.
Active Movement:	Get your heart healthy and strong by doing some exercise that will get your heart pumping. For example, do jumping jacks, high knees, and skip around the room.
Theme Poses:	All of these poses will help open your heart and mind. When introducing them to children, try to follow in this heart opening sequence.

Cat Pose to Cow Pose: Begin on your hands and knees. Next round your back and tuck your chin into your chest as if you are a cat. Then look up, arch your back and open your chest into Cow Pose. This is a great way to begin strengthening your spine and to feel your heart opening.

Updog Pose: Lie on your tummy. Place the palms of your hands next to your shoulders and look up. Slowly straighten your arms and open your chest.

Bridge or Wheel Pose: Kids love trying to get into Wheel Pose, but this huge heart opener is not easily accessible for all. For an easier but still effective heart opener, try Bridge Pose. Lie on your back with your knees bent and your feet flat on the ground. Tilt your chin and lift your chest.

Bow Pose: Lie on your tummy, bend your knees, and lift your chest. Reach your arms back toward your toes and hold onto your feet. Let your heart shine!

Game:	**Web of Love:** This is similar to Human Knot. Children stand in a circle and hold two hands across the circle from them. Try to untangle the group without letting go of hands. The younger the ages, the smaller the group for this game.
Partner/Group Challenge Poses:	**Open Heart:** Each child stands behind their partner with one foot behind them and one foot forward, holding their partner's wrists. The partner in front leans forward and shines his or her heart forward while the other partner helps support them.
Community Closing:	**Heart Mudra:** Children create a heart with their hands. Everyone holds out their heart toward the center of the circle and then rests it at their heart center while sharing what they love most about yoga.
Stillness and Savasana:	Have the children lie down slowly on the ground and wrap their arms around their knees to give themselves a big hug. Next they release into stillness.

Theme:	**Lucky Leprechaun Yoga**
Ages:	3-12
Materials:	Gold coins with the Leprechaun Poses written on them (see themed poses below) and a "pot of gold" bucket or something to hold coins.
Welcome:	What do you know about Leprechauns and St. Patrick's Day?
Breath Work:	**Rainbow Breathing:** Inhale and reach your arms to one side of your body. On the exhale, raise your arms overhead and lower to the other side.
Active Movement:	**Gold Coin Balance Relay:** Divide into two groups. Each person must balance a gold coin on his or her head and deliver it to the pot of gold. See how many coins you can get in the allotted time.
Theme Poses:	Have the children take turns drawing out a gold coin from the bucket as

	they learn the following poses: **Rainbow:** (Wheel Pose) **Pot of Gold:** (Boat Pose) **Leprechaun:** (Chair Pose) Leprechauns are short, happy and light on their feet! Move your head from side to side as if looking for a pot of gold. **Four Leaf Clover:** (Star Pose) **Horseshoe:** (Horse Pose)
Game:	**Irish Jig Freeze:** Play music and dance around the room. When the music stops, freeze into one of the learned yoga poses.
Partner/Group Challenge Poses:	**Pot of Gold Game:** Have children take turns holding a strong Boat Pose. How many gold coins are they able to hold in their "bucket?" Walk around putting the coins into students' buckets.
Community Closing:	**Make a Rainbow:** Make a group rainbow with everyone. See how quickly

	you can do it. Can it be made another way?
Stillness and Savasana:	Be a rainbow fading into your mat or the ground. Lie as still as possible waiting for the next rainstorm.

Theme:	**Ninja Yoga**
Ages:	5-12
Materials:	Hula Hoop
Welcome:	Ninjas are strong, courageous, and silent. What part of their body needs to be strong?
Breath Work:	**Ninja Breath:** Stand up tall with your feet hip distance apart. Inhale and stretch arms up overhead. Then pull down your arms to exhale quickly and say, "Ha."
Sun Salutation:	**Sun A:** Get your body all warmed up and ready by practicing a few sun salutations. Remember your breath.
Active Movement:	Have everyone get in ninja shape by thinking of an exercise they want to do— jumping jacks, push ups, sit-ups, high knees, etc. They also get to select a repetition amount between 1-10. Kids like having a choice in this and most will pick the higher number for their exercise.

Theme Poses:	These poses are all tried and proven to build strength in your whole body.
	Plank Pose
	Warrior 1
	Warrior 2
	Airplane Pose
	Reverse Warrior
	Chair Pose
Game:	**The Ninja Sneak:** Ninjas need to move in all kinds of ways. Practice this by standing in a circle and holding hands with the Hula Hoop. Each person takes a turn moving their body through the hoop without letting go of hands. See if you can make it all the way around the circle.
Partner/Group Challenge Poses:	Build strength in your whole body with Down Dog push ups or have a Plank Pose holding contest.
Community Closing:	Turn the lights down low and take a moment to

	reflect and share on which parts of their body they felt getting stronger while holding these ninja poses.
Stillness and Savasana:	Be as quiet and still as a ninja while you rest in Savasana.

Theme:	**Pirate Yoga Adventure**
Ages:	3-11
Materials:	None
Welcome:	What do you know about pirates?
Breath Work:	**Pirate Breath:** Breathe in deeply through your nose, and on the exhale let out a loud pirate "ARGH!"
Sun Salutation:	**Search for the Treasure Sun A:** On the inhale, sweep your arms up high and look up. On the exhale, swan dive down and search for the treasure below. Repeat several times
Active Movement:	**Walk the Plank** (Follow the Leader): Take turns being the leader and move around the room in different ways. For example, walk on tip-toes, march, walk backward, walk heel to toe, or walk on your heels.
Theme Poses:	**Pirate Boat** (Boat Pose) **Walk the Plank** (Plank Pose) **Parrot** (Airplane Pose) **Treasure Chest** (Cow Pose)

Game:	**Captain Says** (Simon Says): The leader begins by saying "Captain says" or not depending on whether he wants the children to perform the different actions or yoga poses. Examples are pat your head, jump in place, touch toes, do Down Dog Pose, hold Tree Pose, etc.
Partner/Group Challenge Poses: OR Inversion/Balance:	**Double Boat Partner Pose**: Partners sit facing one another with knees bent and toes touching. While holding hands, they lift their legs and go into Boat Pose. To help with balance, the bottoms of their feet should be touching. If the partners are able, they straighten their legs and lean back slightly to make a "V" shape.
Community Closing:	Review the poses they have learned. What other pirate poses can they think of?
Stillness and Savasana:	Even pirates need to rest. Lie down as slowly as you can and take a few moments to be still.

Theme:	**Princess and the Beast**
Ages:	4-12
Breath Work:	**Beast Breath:** Breathe in through your nose. Exhale strongly through your open mouth.
Sun Salutation:	On the inhale, stretch your arms up overhead and make yourself seem really big and towering as if you are the Beast. Then on your exhale, dive forward and bring your hands by your feet. Repeat 3-5 times.
Theme Poses:	**Princess** (Dancer Pose) **Teapot** (Triangle Pose) **Candle** (Shoulder Stand Pose) **Clock** (Duck Pose): Move your head from right to left. **Villain** (Warrior 2 Pose): Face your palm toward yourself as if looking admiringly in the mirror.
Game:	**Servants in the Castle:** Choose one person to be the master. When the

	master has his back turned, all of the castle servants dance and move around. When the master turns back around, everyone must freeze. If the master sees a servant moving, he or she becomes the next master.
Partner/Group Challenge Poses:	**Castle Pose:** Partners work together to create a castle. Stand facing one another with palms touching and outstretched overhead. Each partner takes a step back while keeping their palms touching. See how many times you can take a step back.
Community Closing:	**Circle Showcase:** Everyone shows a favorite pose that they learned.
Stillness and Savasana:	Slowly lower yourself onto your back as if you are a rose slowly losing its petals. Remain in this resting position as still and quiet as possible.

Theme:	**Springtime Yoga**
Ages:	3-12
Materials:	Spring yoga poses (see below) written on slips of paper
Welcome:	What kind of changes happen outside in spring? How do some animals change?
Breath Work:	**Cocoon Breath**: Pretend you are a caterpillar snug in a cocoon. Take deep long breaths in and out as you transform into a butterfly.
Sun Salutation:	You are a flower reaching as high as you can toward the sun. Next dive forward into a forward fold and then stretch up again even taller.
Active Movement:	Have the children be little seeds in the ground. Sprinkle them with water and watch them grow, sometimes very slowly and other times very quickly.
Theme Poses:	**Caterpillar to Butterfly**:

1.   Begin in Cobra Pose. Pretend to be a hungry caterpillar lifting your head to munch on a leaf.

2.   Move into Plank Pose. Now you are the caterpillar on the branch, getting ready to form a cocoon.

3.   Lower yourself into Child's Pose and become a safe little cocoon. Be still. Breathe deeply and get ready for an exciting change to happen.

4.   Finally it is time to become a butterfly! Sit in Butterfly Pose and flutter your wings up and down.

Egg to Tadpole to Frog

1.   Begin in Child's Pose as that represents the tiny egg.

2.   Slowly inch onto your stomach into Superman Pose and move your arms and legs up and down as if you are a tadpole swimming.

3.   Sit in Frog Pose (Malasana Pose) with your feet on the floor and your legs in a deep squat. Try out your new frog legs as you hop around on your mat.

Seed to Flower

	1. Begin in Child's Pose and pretend to be a tiny seed in the ground. 2. Lift one arm as you imagine a tiny stem beginning to poke through the earth. 3. Sit up tall in Lotus Pose with your legs crossed. Raise your arms above your head as if they are petals facing the sun. Can you sway in the breeze?
Game:	**Springtime Yoga Charades**: Have many different spring words written on pieces of paper (ex: tree, flower, bird, rain, sun, frog, caterpillar, bunny, rainbow…) Each student takes a turn drawing one and acting it out with yoga poses for the rest of the class to guess.
Partner/Group Challenge Poses:	**Group Tree**: Stand in a circle in Tree Pose with arms resting on one another's shoulders. See how you are stronger by working together.
Community Closing:	Have each student showcase in the middle of the circle a Spring Pose or transformation that we practiced in

	class or one that they have made up on their own.
Stillness and Savasana:	Pretend you are a tiny seed in the ground. Lie as still as you can while waiting to grow.

Theme:	**Summer Olympics: Go for the Gold!**
Ages:	3-12
Materials:	Music
Welcome:	What are some of your favorite Olympic sports? Why?
Breath Work:	**Floating Feather:** Olympic athletes need to be in control of their breath to help them compete at their top level. Take turns with a partner lying down on a yoga mat. Try to keep your feather afloat with your breath.
Sun Salutation:	**Sun A:** Dive into this sun salutation with your arms outstretched as if you are on the Olympic high diving team.
Active Movement:	**Olympic Boot Camp:** Get your Olympic body strong by doing a series of exercises. Everyone takes a turn picking and leading 10 reps of various exercises such as jumping jacks, hill climbers, push-ups, or squat jumps.

Theme Poses:	**Archery** (Warrior 2): Stand strong in this pose and draw your back arm forward and back as if pulling and releasing your arrow.
	Rowing (Boat Pose): Can you row your arms back and forth as if rowing a boat?
	Arrow Pose (Side Plank with top leg bent and resting on calf)
	Bow Pose (Bow Pose): This is the perfect pose to combine with Arrow Pose.
	Cycling: Do some bicycle crunches while lying on your back. Make your bike go faster and slower
	Taekwondo (Horse Pose): Can you move your arms back and forth with strength as if you are breaking a board?
	Gymnastics (Star Pose Jumps): How high can you jump and stick your landing?
Game:	**Mini Olympics:** Set up a short obstacle course with cones, hoops, or anything

	else you have on hand. Put a yoga pose card between each of the obstacles for the students to perform. Have each student take a turn competing in the Mini Olympics. Time them if you would like.
Partner/Group Challenge Poses:	**Synchronized Swimming:** Place the yoga mats in a line. Lay out a sequence of yoga pose cards in front of each mat. Everyone must perform the poses at the same time. Practice holding each pose for three breaths. This is more challenging than it sounds!
Community Closing:	Have each student showcase a favorite pose and announce if they won a Gold Medal by doing the best they can.
Stillness and Savasana:	Rest and relax your Olympic body on the mat. You deserve it!

Theme:	**Theme Park Fun**
Ages:	3-10
Welcome:	What kinds of things would you see at an amusement park? Which food or rides?
Breath Work:	**Balloon Breath:** Inhale and bring your arms up and out to your side creating a large balloon. Then on the exhale let your balloon go while bringing your hands back to heart center.
Sun Salutation:	**Ferris Wheel:** Bend over in Ragdoll Pose with elbows grasped. Breathe in and reach your arms in a circle as if you are riding on a Ferris Wheel.
Active Movement:	**Pop Popcorn:** Hug your knees and squeeze your body into a tight ball like a popcorn kernel. When you get nice and hot, jump into the air as if you are popping. **Lemonade Stand:** Roll back and forth on your yoga mat as if you are a

	lemon rolling. Then sit up and squeeze your legs tightly as if you squeezing a lemon and making lemonade. Then release all of the muscles in your body.
Theme Poses:	**Pretzel Pose:** (Lotus Pose) Sit cross-legged. Take each foot and place it on the opposite thigh. **Carousel:** (Horse Pose) Can you make your horse move up and down as if on a carousel? **Giant Slide:** (Reverse Plank Pose) Sit with your legs straight out in front of you. Point your toes as you lift your hips. Relax your head and neck.
Game:	**Ride the Roller Coaster:** Everyone sits closely in a line and spreads their legs in a "V" shape. Act as if you are heading up a hill and lean back. Then move forward as if going down the hill. Lean left and right as if going around curves.

Partner/Group Challenge Poses:	**Down Dog Tunnel:** Make your own ride with this pose. Everyone goes into Down Dog next to one another. Begin with the child on the end and have him or her crawl through and then resume Down Dog Pose on the other side. Continue on until everyone has made it through.
Community Closing:	What was your favorite part of class?
Stillness and Savasana:	**Corn Dog Pose:** Lie on your yoga mat. With your arms at your side, pull up the edges of the mat to make a hot dog bun.

Theme:	**Welcome Winter**
Ages:	3-12
Materials:	Music
Welcome:	What is your favorite thing about Winter? Why?
Breathwork:	Breathe in and out through your open mouth as if you are fogging up a window.
Sun Salutation:	**Make it Snow!** Breathe into Mountain Pose with arms out stretched to the sky. Now dive forward as if you are a snowflake landing to the ground. Repeat while using your breath.
Active Movement:	Go sledding with your yoga mat. Have the children sit cross legged near the front of their mats and hold onto the top. Rock and roll on the mat while hanging on.
Theme Poses:	**Holiday Tree** (Tree Pose) **Ice Skater** (Airplane Pose) **Reindeer** (Chair Pose) **Sleigh** (Boat Pose) **Gingerbread Man** (Star Pose)

Game:	**Freeze Dance:** Dance around the room. When the music stops, everyone freezes into a favorite yoga pose they just learned.
Partner/Group Challenge Poses:	**Sleigh Ride:** Each child sits on floor with legs in front of them with a "V" shape. The next child sits directly in front of them. Announce that we need everyone's help to get the sleigh off the ground. Each student says, "Heave" and leans forward. Then say, "Heave Ho" and lean back. Keep this going by working together.
Community Closing:	**Sharing Circle:** Let each student take a turn sharing a word or phrase that describes how they are feeling at this moment at the end of class. Often times I am surprised at the insightfulness of the students as they relay words of calm, peace, content, strong, relaxed…This exercise helps promote a good feeling of self-awareness, peace and empathy toward others. They are simple words, but they are powerful in carrying that

	feeling and awareness outside of class.
Stillness and Savasana:	Pretend you are a snowflake falling from the sky. Be as still as you can as you lightly land on the ground and stay.

Chapter 11: Quick and Easy No-Time-to-Plan Kids Yoga Lesson

Admittedly, I am a planner, and I hope the lesson plans laid out in this book provide you with a good variety of yoga poses, games, and activities for teaching yoga to children. What happens if you find yourself in a pinch, and there is no time to plan for a kids yoga class? Or maybe you have only a few moments and really want to make the most of that time at school or at home with your children? No problem.

Introducing yoga to children doesn't always need to include a full theme that is planned out from beginning to end. Children can still experience the fun and receive the benefits of yoga in a quick 10-20 minute session. It is almost like an express class, and it is definitely effective when you only have a few moments to spare. This lesson is perfect for use at home, school, or in a studio.

Our Go-To Kids Yoga Express Plan can work with any children age three and up. With a few materials, this kids yoga lesson plan will have your students engaged and learning while getting fit and flexible.

1. Breathe

I like to begin with the children in a circle as it creates a feeling of community. Do a few breathing exercises together to help unite the class in breath. There are dozens of breathing exercises in this book or in *Go Go Yoga for Kids a Complete Guide for Using Yoga with Kids*. This can be as simple as practicing Balloon Breath. Breathe in and extend arms overhead. Then breathe out and bring hands to heart center. Do several times. This one is definitely a go-to favorite of kids.

2. Move

Shake the wiggles out, get hearts pumping, and warm up the body with some movement. Keep it simple with sun salutations or have the children do some exercises such as push-ups, jumping jacks, or high knees. Gauge your students. If they have been sitting all day in school then they will definitely be ready for some big movements. I have found that after spending a few moments on large motor movement, the children are much more attentive for the rest of class. It is almost as if they have re-awoken their brains and bodies.

3. Learn

Select four to five pose cards from the *Kids Yoga Challenge Pose Cards* and place them in a bag for the students to draw from. Using a bag or prop to hold the cards creates anticipation and lets the children feel like they have some sort of choice or control in which card is selected.

Select one quiet listener to choose a pose card from your bag. He or she places the pose card in the center of the circle. Demonstrate the pose and have everyone practice it. Select another child to choose a pose from the bag. Continue with this until all poses have been introduced.

Page 108

4. Flow

The pose cards are already in the center of the circle. Turn on music and have everyone hold the pose for two to three breaths before continuing on to the next pose.

Kids love this as they are able to practice and then master the poses. They also feel their poses differently in their body as their bodies warm up. I also tell the students that this is similar to an adult class where they learn the poses and then put them into a flow. I usually play upbeat or familiar music from a recent kid movie.

5. Recover

After the Yoga Flow, have the students go into Child's Pose or sit comfortably for a few moments to catch their breath and re-center themselves. Congratulate them on a job well done.

6. Shine

Have each child take a moment to be the Yoga Star by going to the center of the circle and showing off their favorite pose. Have them demonstrate kindness and mindfulness for their fellow classmates as they each take a turn.

7. Rest

Challenge the children to lie down as slowly as they can as if they are an icicle melting. Allow them to lie down however they feel comfortable—on their back or side or stomach for Savasana. Play relaxing music for a few moments. Thirty seconds to a minute is a reasonable amount of time at this age for children to be able to practice stillness.

8. Ready

Slowly have the children sit up. Lead them in a few cleansing breaths together as a group. They can do this by moving their arms overhead and exhaling out as they bring their hands to heart center. Close your class with a thoughtful and encouraging message that they can carry with them for the rest of their day. Namaste.

Chapter 12: Read Aloud Books for Yoga and Movement

If you are a teacher, parent, counselor, or you work with children in any way, this part is especially important for you to remember as you interact with children. Anyone can read aloud to kids and help them benefit mentally and physically.

As a teacher and reading specialist, I understand the power of reading aloud to children and the great number of benefits that accompany it. By combining reading aloud with yoga poses, you have children who are becoming mindful, fit, and literate.

I have noticed as a parent and during my twenty plus years of working with children, how deeply touched they are by the books they read or listen to. One of my favorite things to do in my school classroom, kids yoga class, or at home with my own children is to read aloud. Books provide the opportunity to teach important life lessons. Children relate to books and the lessons taught in them in a way that is powerful and memorable.

Children who are read aloud to get a head start in language and literacy. It increases their vocabulary and opportunity for comprehension practice. When combined with yoga, children will be moving and stretching their bodies, increasing their focus and balance, and having fun!

When kids are moving, it helps them enhance their understanding and retention of what they have learned. This is called kinesthetic learning, and it is perfect to use with those busy, wiggly kids who need to move their bodies during or after those long school days of sitting.

How to Use these Read Aloud Yoga Lesson Plans

There are many books by respected authors who have recognized the need to share important topics with tomorrow's leaders. The following lesson plans include quality children's literature that is popular, fun to read aloud, and provides opportunity for movement. These books could be part of a curriculum at school such as the ocean, ABC's, or the rainforest, but they do not have to be. They can also stand alone to provide an important message or lesson.

The following books are also wonderful additions to read aloud at home with children. With the included poses and movement, they will especially enjoy, remember, and retain these books.

How to Use These Books with Children:

All the lesson plans include a Creating a Connection component. This allows you to help the children make a connection before you read the book. By asking these questions and letting the students answer, it activates their prior knowledge and also allows them to connect with the story. They will better remember the story by doing this.

Each lesson plan includes an underlying theme that can be emphasized and taught. The lesson plan also includes breathing exercises that correspond with the book. By incorporating these simple breathing exercises, you will be giving children tools to help them be calm and mindful.

After creating a connection, read the book aloud and let the children enjoy the story and become familiar with the characters. This will provide a greater understanding as you next incorporate movement and yoga poses.

All of the yoga poses listed for each book help connect the story to movement. If you are unsure of what the pose looks like, please refer to the Pose Glossary at the end of this book.

First, read the story. Then on subsequent readings incorporate the yoga poses and movement. The yoga poses also provide a wonderful way to act out and retell the story.

Finally, each lesson plan includes relaxation or stillness exercises, which allows the children to practice being still, calm, and mindful. By including this stillness at the end of the story, you are providing an idea as well as an opportunity to transition into the next activity.

Title: *The Giving Tree*	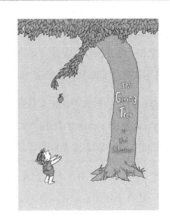
Author: Shel Silverstein	
Theme: Generosity and thinking of others before yourself	

Creating a Connection:

What kind of things can you give to others that don't cost anything? Hugs, smiles, and high fives are all completely free and make others feel happy. *The Giving Tree* by Shel Silverstein is about a tree that gave and gave to someone he loved most.

Breath Work:

We all need to give our bodies something all the time to help them stay healthy, strong, and happy. It is completely free and doesn't cost a thing. Does anyone know what that is? Our breath. Practice breathing in to the count of three through your nose and then out through your nose.

Read Aloud:

Read the book aloud and pause to comment on the different ways the tree is helping the boy.

Poses:

Child's Pose: The boy is a child in the beginning of the book.

Tree Pose: Stand strong and tall in tree pose.

Movement:

Have the students move or dance around the room to music. When the leader calls out a number between 1-20, that is the number of breaths everyone needs to take while in Tree Pose. This is a great activity to work on balance and focus.

Stillness:

Become like the old man and the tree at the end of the book. Sit or lie down on your back or side, whatever feels comfortable, and rest.

Title: *Where the Wild Things Are*	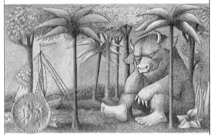
Author: Maurice Sendak	
Theme: Working through anger or frustration	

Creating a Connection:

Have the children share how they are feeling right now at this moment (happy, nervous, hungry, tired, excited, sad). Ask why they are feeling that way. Explain that in the book *Where the Wild Things Are,* Max is upset with his mom. Ask the children to think about a time they were upset or mad at their mom, dad, brother, sister, or someone else. Have the children close their eyes and reflect briefly about that time. How did it make them feel? Where in their body did they feel this emotion? Stomach, head, heart?

Breath Work:

We all need a way to get rid of angry feelings or to calm down. We are going to blow these angry feelings away with our breath. On the count of five, breathe in through your nose, and then exhale out strongly through your mouth. Practice this a few times.

Read Aloud:

Read the book aloud. Pause to comment on the wild
things in the book and what can be done to calm them.

Poses:

Where the Wild Things Are is an excellent book to work
on poses that open up your heart and allow yourself to be
peaceful and calm.

Cat Pose to Cow Pose: Begin on all fours and alternate
between the poses. Be sure to use sounds or breathe as
you transition between the poses.

Updog Pose: This pose truly allows for your heart to
shine.

Bridge Pose: Raise your heart up in this lying- down
position and let it be the highest part of your body.

Wheel Pose: This advanced heart-opener pose is not for
everyone, but after completing the poses above, your
body is more ready for it.

Movement:

Have your own Wild Rumpus. Turn the lights down low
and play some music. When the music stops, have
everyone freeze into their favorite pose.

Stillness:

Welcome back from the Wild Rumpus. It is now time to
rest just like Max in the book. Lie or sit comfortably and
allow your body to be still and mindful.

Title: *Commotion in the Ocean*	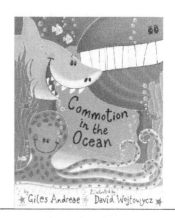
Author: Giles Andreae and David Wojtowycz	
Theme: Learn about the animals that live in the ocean.	

Creating a Connection:

What animals live in the ocean? Which ones are your favorites?

Breath Work:

Breathe in and out deeply making the sound of ocean waves crashing to shore on your exhale.

Read Aloud:

Read the book aloud enjoying the rhyme and illustrations with the children.

Poses:

Dolphin Pose: Can you squeak and be playful like a dolphin?

Shark (Bow Pose): Make a fin with your hands on your back

Jellyfish (Ragdoll Pose): Let your arms hang and jiggle like a jellyfish.

Boat Pose: Row your boat back and forth through the ocean.

Movement:

The Beach Towel Scramble game requires each child to have their own spot on the carpet or around the room. Play some music and allow the children to move or dance around the room. When the music stops, find a beach towel or special spot to hold a yoga pose. Continue again.

Stillness:

Become like a starfish and lie down peacefully in the sand.

Title: *Rumble in the Jungle*	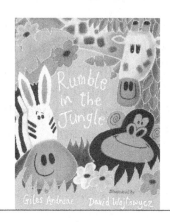
Author: Giles Andreae and David Wojtowycz	
Theme: Learn about the animals who live in the jungle.	

Creating a Connection:

What animals live in the jungle? What noises do they make?

Breath Work:

Practice Snake Breath by breathing in through your nose. On the exhale, make a large hissing sound as you pretend to be a snake.

Read Aloud:

Read the book aloud enjoying the rhyme and illustrations with the children.

Poses:

Bend at your waist and place your palms underneath your feet to make Gorilla Pose.

Giraffe (Tree Pose): Extend your arms above your head.

Cobra (Updog Pose): Hiss like a snake.

Elephant (One-armed Down Dog): Swing your "trunk" from side to side.

Movement:

Go on a jungle adventure: Pretend to move like different animals in the jungle would. Lumber like a bear, swing through the trees as if you are a monkey, and slither on your tummy like a snake.

Stillness:

Lie comfortably on your back, tummy, or side and listen to the relaxing sound of rain in the jungle.

Title: *Pete the Cat*	
Author: Eric Litwin	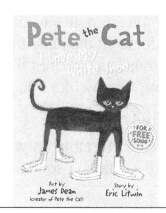
Theme: Be content with what you have, be positive, and do not take things too seriously.	

Creating a Connection:
What is one of your favorite things? In this book Pete the Cat has some new shoes, and he is very proud of them. But something happens to his shoes. Notice how he reacts when things go wrong.

Breath Work:
Practice Lion's Breath by breathing in through your nose. On the exhale, stick out your tongue and saying "ahhh."

Read Aloud:
Read the book aloud to the children. They will enjoy the catchy rhyme and series of events that Pete goes through with his new white shoes.

Poses: **Cat Pose to Cow Pose** **Down Dog Pose**
Movement:

Follow the leader. Take turns being the leader and have everyone follow what the leader is doing such as walk on tip toes, walk backwards, pat head, Cat Pose, walk the dog in Down Dog Pose, etc.

Stillness: Take a quiet catnap.

Title: *Angry Octopus*	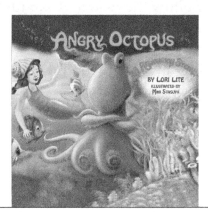
Author: Lori Lite	
Theme: Learn to be calm and to manage stress and anxiety.	

Creating a Connection:

When was a time you felt angry? What did you do? In *Angry Octopus*, the octopus feels overwhelmed and anxious. Notice how he reacts.

Breath Work:

This whole book is wonderful for introducing children to the importance of taking deep breaths and being calm. Have the children practice taking deep breaths in through their nose and out their mouth.

Read Aloud:

Enjoy reading the book aloud to children and discussing how to be the boss of your own body and emotions.

Poses:

Octopus (Ragdoll Pose): Bend at the waist and allow your arms to dangle and move as if you are an octopus with eight legs.

Sea Child (Updog Pose): Can you tilt your head from left to right?

Movement:

The game Octopus Tag requires room to move and run. Select one child to be the octopus. The octopus is allowed to run anywhere in the room. The rest of the children line up along the wall. When the child says "Octopus," the children all run from one side of the room to the other. Anyone the octopus touches becomes the seaweed. They need to stay in the spot they were tagged, but they can use their arms to tag others. If others are tagged, they become the seaweed as well.

Stillness:

Be like the octopus and lie down on your back, close your eyes, and take a deep breath. Breathe in through your nose and let the air out of your mouth…ahhh. Guide the children through the relaxation exercise given in the book.

Title: *Downward Mule*	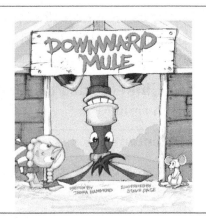
Author: Jenna Hammond	
Theme: Learn the importance of being yourself.	

Creating a Connection:

What animals live on a farm? When was a time that you felt different or that you didn't really fit in or belong? How did that make you feel?

Breath Work:

In this book, the donkey feels calm and peaceful as he breathes deeply in and out of his mouth. Practice the same breathing exercise that the donkey does.

Read Aloud:

Enjoy reading the book aloud to children. They will enjoy the familiar barnyard animals.

Poses:

This entire book leads to movement and poses. Enjoy reading the book aloud, but pause and allow the children to practice the poses. A few poses include: Cat Pose, Crow Pose, Cow Pose, Down Dog Pose, and Tree Pose.

Movement:

To practice donkey kicks, begin in Down Dog Pose and begin to kick your heels to the sky. Be mindful of those around you.

Stillness:

This story provides an opportunity for stillness and relaxation at the end. Breathe in, breathe out, and watch the clouds above.

Title: *Chicka Chicka Boom Boom*	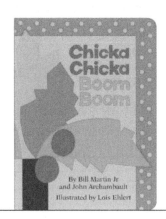
Author: Bill Martin Jr.	
Theme: Even if you fall or things get hard, get back up and keep trying your best.	

Creating a Connection:

Use the alphabet chart at the beginning of the book, and practice saying the alphabet together. Change it up by speaking in pirate voices or squeaky mouse voices. This keeps all the children engaged.

Breath Work:

The sun rises and sets in this book. Practice a few sun salutations by raising your arms above your head and then diving forward with arms outstretched. Remember to breathe in as you rise up and breathe out as you fold.

Read Aloud:

This book includes catchy rhymes. Have the children join in when they can with special attention to the 'Chicka Chicka Boom Boom' lines.

Poses:

While in Tree Pose, can you raise your hands above you and make fists as if they are coconuts?

Movement:

To make Alphabet Soup, have the children practice forming different letters with their bodies. Begin with letters that are formed easily such as I, O, and T. Then see what letters they can create. There are no right or wrong answers. This is a wonderful way for children to move and practice the alphabet.

Stillness:

Be still and sleep like the letters at the end of the book.

Title: *I Am Yoga*	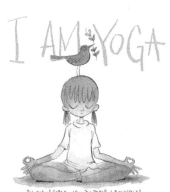
Author: Susan Verde	
Theme:	
You can be anything you set your mind to. Yoga calms and strengthens our minds, but with a little imagination anything is possible.	

Creating a Connection:

What does yoga mean? Talk with the children about yoga being a form of exercise. Yoga makes you feel good inside and out.

Breath Work:

Explain to the children that yoga begins with breath. If you aren't breathing, you aren't doing yoga. Get your body ready for yoga by breathing in through your nose for the count of three, holding your breath, and then breathing out for the count of three.

Read Aloud:

Enjoy reading the book aloud and notice the illustrations and how the book makes them feel.

Poses:

Try the variety of poses that are given and demonstrated in the book.

Movement:

Have each child select a favorite pose. It can be a yoga pose or one that they made up. Stand in a circle. Have them state their name, demonstrate a favorite yoga pose, and mention a characteristic about themselves.

For example, "I am Sara. I am strong." I would then stand in Warrior 2 Pose. The rest of the children and leader would respond, "This is Sara. She is strong," as they also stand in Warrior 2 Pose. Continue around the circle with everyone getting a turn. It is wonderful to see what poses the children select and what they say about themselves. If they need help selecting a pose, be sure to have the *Kids Yoga Challenge Pose Cards* or other yoga pose cards for children to model so they do not feel stuck.

Stillness: Choose a comfortable position on your back, side, or stomach. Breathe and be still.

Title: *I Am Peace*	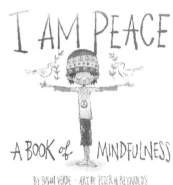
Author: Susan Verde	
Theme:	
Mindfulness means being fully engaged in the present moment. Practice learning how to be peaceful, present, and mindful in the moment you are in.	

Creating a Connection:

What does being peaceful or mindful mean? Brainstorm together about ways that you can show mindfulness to others at home or school

Breath Work:

Place your hand in front of your mouth and notice your breath. Is it warm or cool? Just notice as you take big breaths in and out.

Read Aloud:

Read aloud *I Am Peace*. Enjoy the beautiful illustrations and message about demonstrating peace.

Poses:

Practice these peaceful poses.

Child's Pose: Bring your forehead to the floor and breathe deeply.

Lotus Pose: Bring your hands to heart center.

Reverse Warrior: Gaze at your hand above your head in this peaceful pose.

Movement:

"I can" is a phrase that is repeated frequently in the story. Have the children stand in a circle and take a moment to say something that they can do along with a corresponding movement. For example, "I can touch my toes," or "I can reach up to the sky."

Stillness:

Practice mindful breathing by either lying down or finding a comfortable position and closing your eyes. Place your hands on your belly. Notice your breathing. Is it fast or slow? Begin to breathe through your nose and notice how that slows your breathing down and how you become more calm and relaxed.

Title: *The Very Hungry Caterpillar* **Author:** Eric Carle	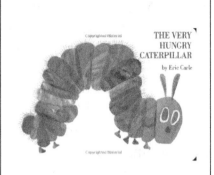

Theme:

We are all growing and changing. In this story we are taken through the life cycle of a caterpillar as he becomes a butterfly.

Creating a Connection:

What happens to a caterpillar? Discuss briefly about what a caterpillar needs to do in order to become a butterfly.

Breath Work:

Pretend you are in a little cocoon and must breathe deeply to be able to emerge as a butterfly.

Read Aloud:

Children love this story as they recognize the days of the week and the different foods.

Poses:

Go through each of these poses to represent the life cycle of a caterpillar.

Egg: (Child's Pose)

Caterpillar: (Locust Pose)

Cocoon: (Plank Pose)

Butterfly: (Butterfly Pose)

Movement:

Practice retelling the story adding the yoga poses and movement together to act out the story.

Stillness:

If you are using yoga mats, roll each child up in a cocoon with their yoga mat. If you are not using mats, children can roll themselves up into a tight little ball.

Title: *The Great Kapok Tree*	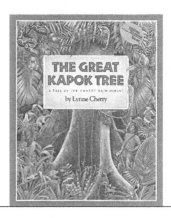
Author: Lynne Cherry	
Theme: Learn the importance of trees and how to care for the environment. All living things depend on one another.	

Creating a Connection:

Why are trees important? What do people and animals use trees for?

Breath Work:

All living things, including trees, need oxygen to stay alive. Practice taking deep breaths in and out through you nose.

Read Aloud:

Read aloud *The Great Kapok Tree* and notice how many animals depend on this tree for survival.

Poses:

Go through each of these poses to represent parts of this story. Discuss what their reasons were for not wanting the tree chopped down.

The Kapok Tree: Tree Pose

Boa Constrictor: Updog Pose

Monkey: Gorilla Pose

Macaw: Airplane Pose

Tree Frog: Malasana Pose

Jaguar: Chair Pose

Porcupine: Cat Pose to Cow Pose

Sloth: Child's Pose

Movement:

Practice retelling the story adding the yoga poses and movement together to act out the story.

Stillness:

Be as still as the man sleeping during the story when each of the animals visits him.

Yoga Bingo is a fun game to play with children of all ages.
Download six full-color printable Bingo cards at
http://www.gogoyogakids.com/bingo/

Y	O	G	A
Cat Pose	Cow Pose	Mountain Pose	Shoulder Stand
Down Dog	Updog	Chair Pose	Boat Pose
Plank Pose	Wheel Pose	Warrior 1	Bow Pose
Child's Pose	Triangle Pose	Bridge Pose	Dolphin Pose

Chapter 13: Pose Glossary

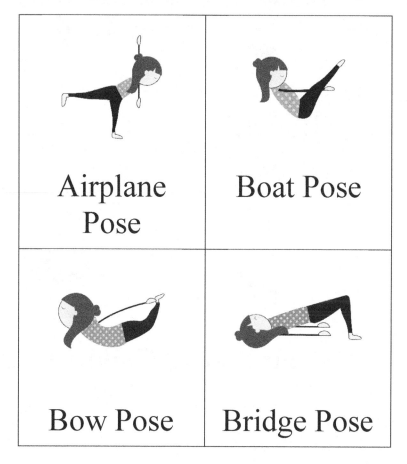

| Airplane Pose | Boat Pose |
| Bow Pose | Bridge Pose |

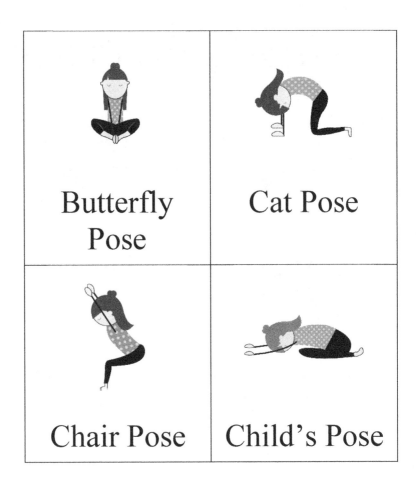

Butterfly Pose	Cat Pose
Chair Pose	Child's Pose

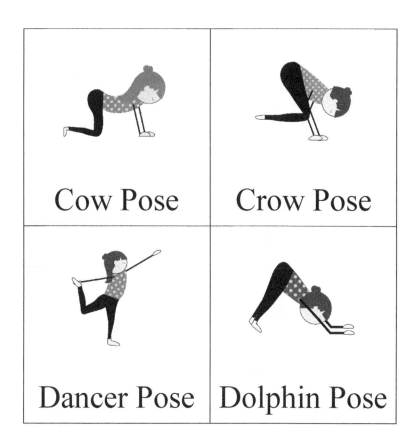

Cow Pose	Crow Pose
Dancer Pose	Dolphin Pose

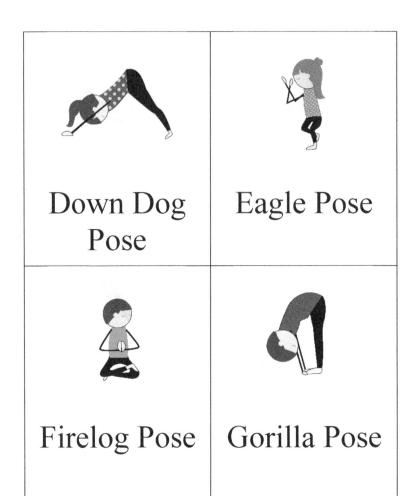

| Down Dog Pose | Eagle Pose |
| Firelog Pose | Gorilla Pose |

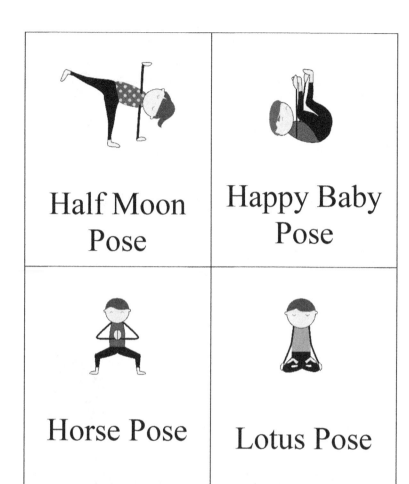

| Half Moon Pose | Happy Baby Pose |
| Horse Pose | Lotus Pose |

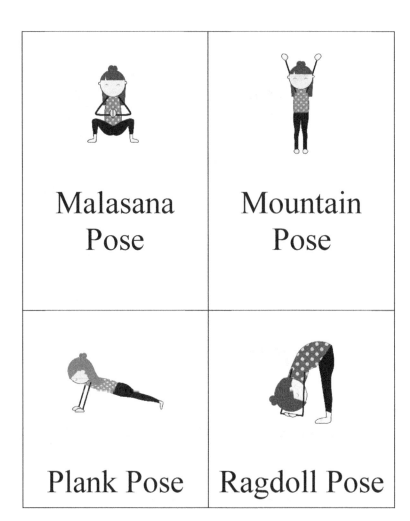

Malasana Pose	Mountain Pose
Plank Pose	Ragdoll Pose

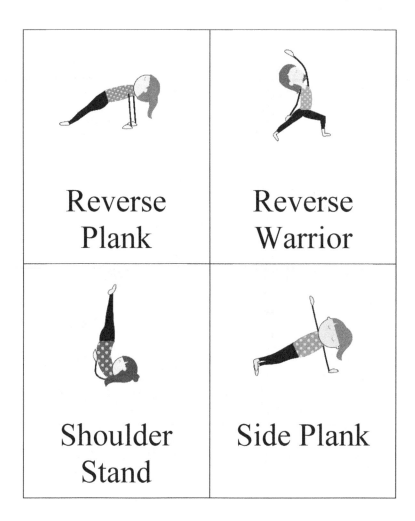

| Reverse Plank | Reverse Warrior |
| Shoulder Stand | Side Plank |

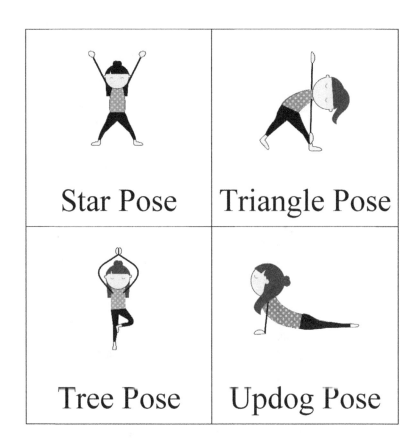

Star Pose	Triangle Pose
Tree Pose	Updog Pose

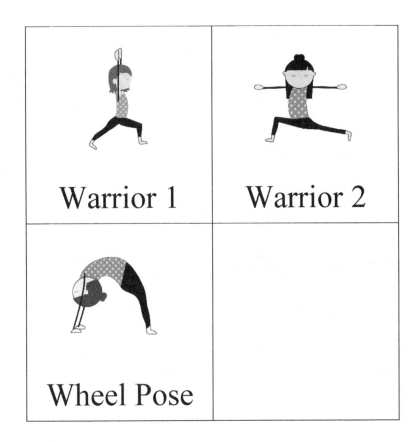

| Warrior 1 | Warrior 2 |
| Wheel Pose | |

About the Author

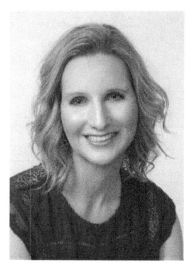

Best-selling author Sara J. Weis is a creative and passionate teacher that has inspired children in and out of the classroom for over twenty years. Through *Go Go Yoga for Kids* she has combined her experience as an elementary teacher and certified kid and adult yoga instructor to help introduce children to the lifelong benefits of yoga.

Sara is passionate about introducing children to yoga in child friendly ways because yoga has so many mental and physical benefits. She is the author of *Go Go Yoga for Kids: A Complete Guide to Using Yoga with Kids*, creator of the *Kids Yoga Challenge Pose Cards* and The Kids Yoga Challenge App. Sara has also taught over 3,000 adults how to successfully teach yoga and mindfulness to children in her online Kids Yoga and Mindfulness Teacher Training.

Sara holds a master's degree in education as well as a bachelor's degree in early childhood and elementary education. She has invested countless hours creating and leading yoga classes for thousands of children. Sara feels strongly about having all of the ideas, strategies, and lessons in one place so that anyone who works with kids will be able to introduce yoga to children with confidence and success.

Sara is a classroom teacher and leads kids yoga classes for a nationally known health and fitness club. She lives in Iowa with her husband, three children, and yoga pup, Rocky.

Thank you for your interest in learning to teach yoga and mindfulness to children. Be sure to download your free Yoga Pose Bingo Cards at gogoyogakids.com/bingo

Please connect with us at the following places.

	http://www.gogoyogakids.com/
	http://www.facebook.com/gogoyogakids/
	http://www.pinterest.com/gogoyogakids/
	http://www.twitter.com/gogoyogakids/
	http://www.instagram.com/gogoyogakids/
	http://www.gogoyogakids.com/youtube/
	The Kids Yoga Challenge Pose Cards http://www.gogoyogakids.com/cards/
	Go Go Yoga for Kids: A Complete Guide to Yoga with Kids http://www.gogoyogakids.com/amazon/

	The Kids Yoga Challenge App http://www.gogoyogakids.com/app/
	The Kids Yoga and Mindfulness Online Teacher Training https://training.gogoyogakids.com/

Index

affirmations 41

airplane pose.... 23, 34, 38, 45, 57, 70, 73, 88, 90, 104, 137, 139

Angry Octopus 124

balance...36, 38, 111

ball...30, 31, 37, 135

Ball Pass 30

balloon breath 63, 101

beanbags 36

beast breath...92

belly breathing...15

benefits 6, 107

bingo cards 23

birthday candle 15

boat pose............... 20, 70, 76, 79, 85, 90, 91, 99, 104, 118, 139

body scan...43, 44

bow pose 58, 68, 82, 99, 118, 139

breathe 108

Breathing Ball 37

breathing buddies 17, 36

breathing exercises 7, 10, 15, 35, 45, 112

breathwork...15, 17

bridge pose 82, 117, 139

butterfly pose...95, 135, 140

camp 14

candle breath 63

cat pose............... 10, 19, 23, 53, 54, 82, 117, 122, 126, 137, 140

chair pose............... 58, 65, 73, 76, 85, 88, 104, 140

Chicka Chicka Boom Boom...128

child's pose............ 19, 70, 95, 96, 109, 115, 132, 134, 137, 140

Choose Your Pose 25

classroom...31

cobra pose...95
Commotion in the Ocean..118
community building 37
community closing 13
cow pose.................. 10, 19, 53, 82, 90, 117, 122, 126, 137, 141
crow pose...126, 141
dancer pose......................... 24, 34, 36, 45, 61, 92, 141
dolphin pose 118, 141
down dog pose 19, 26, 53, 55, 60, 77, 79, 88, 91, 103, 120, 122, 126, 127, 142
down dog tunnel.............................59, 71, 80, 103
downward dog tunnels 22
Downward Mule...126
dragon's breath...17
drishti..45
dry erase board 38
eagle pose 57, 142
emotions 43, 45
express plan 107
family 14
feathers 35
firelog pose 79, 142
flow..109
focal point...38, 45
forward fold...24
freeze dance...105
Go Go Yoga for Kids: A Complete Guide to Using Yoga with Kids 2
gorilla pose 137, 142
group challenges..40
half moon pose 73, 79, 143
happy baby pose 143
happy birthday...65
Head, Shoulders, Knees, and Toes Yoga 24
heart mudra...83

Hoberman Sphere 17, 37

home 5, 14, 111, 112

horse pose 53, 85, 99, 102, 143

Hula Hoop 87

Hula Hoop Tunnel 24

hula hoops 38

human knot 83

I Am Peace 132

I Am Yoga 130

Instinct 33

Invent a Pose 28

Inversion/Balance Work 13

jump ropes 38

Jump the Mats 25

Kids Yoga Challenge Pose Cards .. 2, 18, 21, 22, 23, 25, 26, 27, 30, 32, 33, 34, 36, 41, 108, 131

kids yoga class 47

kids yoga teacher training 2

lesson plans 2, 5, 9, 10, 12, 13, 18, 47, 112, 113

lion's breath 54, 60, 122

literature 13

Literature Books 37

locust pose 135

lotus pose 73, 96, 102, 132, 143

malasana pose 95, 137, 144

mantras 40, 41

meditation 10, 39

mindful 112, 113, 117, 127, 133

mindfulness 5, 9, 10, 32, 33, 37, 40, 43, 45, 132

mindfulness jar 45

mountain pose 20, 33, 34, 72, 104, 144

movement 112, 113

moving meditation 40, 41

musical mats 27

Noisy Bell/Quiet Bell 32

ocean breath...67
open heart 83
partner pose 40, 91
Partner/Group Poses..13
pass the squeeze 59
Pete the Cat...122
pinwheel breath 17
pirate breath...90
plank pose 9, 73, 88, 90, 95, 135, 144
plow pose...31
Plow Race..31
pom-pom balls..28, 35
Pose of the Week..33
ragdoll pose 20, 58, 101, 118, 125, 144
read aloud..112
read aloud books...13, 111
Read Alouds 37
reverse plank 145
reverse plank pose 64, 76, 102
reverse warrior...42, 88, 133, 145
Ring Around the Yogi...23
Rock/Tree/Bridge Relay...26
roller coaster breath..16
rope walk 39
Rumble in the Jungle...120
savasana..13, 109
school 14, 111, 112
School Based Yoga Games 31
seasonal item 39
shoulder stand...145
shoulder stand pose 64, 65, 76, 92
side plank...99, 145
snowflake breathing 16
star pose..................... 61, 65, 70, 73, 85, 99, 104, 146
stillness..113, 127

Page 155

straw breathing 16
sun salutations 41, 128
templates..47
The Giving Tree 114
The Great Kapok Tree..136
The Very Hungry Caterpillar 134
Toega..28, 35
Top 9 Yoga Poses for Kids 19
tree pose...... 20, 33, 34, 36, 38, 45, 68, 70, 73, 91, 96, 104, 115,
    120, 126, 128, 136, 146
triangle breath...16
triangle pose 23, 24, 79, 92, 146
updog pose.................... 19, 55, 60, 82, 117, 120, 125, 136, 146
warrior 1 ....9, 42, 88, 147
warrior 2 .... 42, 67, 88, 92, 99, 131, 147
wheel pose 82, 85, 117, 147
Where the Wild Things Are 116
Yoga Bingo 23
Yoga Dice Game 26
yoga games 18, 21, 38
yoga lesson plans...112
yoga mat 104, 135
yoga obstacle course...39
Yoga Pictures 30, 38
yoga poses 18, 23, 27, 36, 39, 40, 41, 113
yoga props 35
Yoga Queen...22
yoga sandwich 76
Yoga Show 27
yoga star 109
yoga studios...14
Yoga Twister..29

Made in United States
Orlando, FL
31 October 2023

38451383R00088